I had been in pain most of my life I had chronic fatigue and couldn't get through a day .... and connective tissues ached, and my tendons felt raw all the time.

I had allergies and thyroid problems, and had been a jaw-clencher for more than 16 years. Sometimes it felt like my jaw muscles were cramping 24 hours a day. I wore a mouth guard at night and took dentist-prescribed muscle-relaxers to help with my jaw cramping, but who wants to live their whole life on prescription drugs?

I was wondering, "What kind of life is this?"

After my first two visits with Dr. Rodriguez, my body felt better than it had in years. My headache and jaw ache were gone. I had more energy. I actually went through the week following my second visit with him without taking a nap. It had been at least five years since I could do that.

Now, four months after I began treating with Dr. Rodriguez, my overall health is much better and continually improving. My allergies are under much better control, my jaw-clenching has decreased dramatically, my digestive issues are healing, and my joints and tendons no longer ache. Instead of taking afternoon naps, I work extra hours! I feel better than I have in a long time.

— **Karen F.**

Before I started going to Dr. Abel, another doctor told me that my thyroid was flat-lined, I had malabsorption, leaky gut syndrome, and was on the fast track to the autoimmune disease fibromyalgia. I am an energy healer myself. I knew from my work that emotions are the core cause, and that too much stress for too many years can cause thyroid problems, but I had not been able to isolate my exact cause.

Abel cleared all of my core emotional issues in a week and a half. I felt amazing! I weaned off all medication (on my own advice). I don't have any more digestive issues. I'm totally off the thyroid medication I had been taking for 20 years.

Now I don't even go to Abel's office. I just call him and he heals me over the phone. Dr. Abel has greatly, greatly gifted me.

— **Christina Rose**

My son was diagnosed as autistic. He didn't speak the entire two years he was in preschool. He had a really hard time in first grade, as he still wasn't speaking much. If something bothered him, he would just shut down and not speak for two to four hours. He didn't even smile or laugh.

I took him to professionals who told me, "He won't get better. You don't get well from autism."

When my son was 8 or 9 years old, I started going to Dr. Rodriguez for some minor health issues of my own. One day I mentioned my son, who was at home at the time. Dr. Rodriguez treated him remotely, using my arm as the surrogate for his muscle testing.

My son starting getting better that first week. He began smiling and laughing for the first time in his life.

Over time, maybe 1 or 1½ years of sporadic treatments from Dr. Rodriguez, my son began communicating instead of shutting down. He can actually hold a conversation now and lets me know how he's feeling. He'll ask what something means if he doesn't understand, and sometimes he even asks how I am feeling. It's amazing. I always knew he was in there somewhere. I am very grateful.

— **Angela Roosevelt**

Three years ago, I wasn't doing so well. I was very depressed and anxious, and I had a lot of neck and back pain and muscle aches. I was on the edge and felt like giving up. I didn't know what to do. Then I came across Dr. Abel's flyer and decided to try his energy healing.

It took me about two or three visits to begin believing in what he does. After the third visit, I felt some major changes. I went consistently, twice a week, and got better and better and better. In a couple of months, I didn't have to see him as often, only once every three to five weeks. Then I got down to once every four to six months for tune-ups.

Abel genuinely cares about healing people, and helping them get better. The work that he does is life changing. What he did for me is a miracle. He saved my life.

— **Phi Lam**

I had quite a few long-term health problems. My digestion was really, really bad. I was able to eat only 10 or 12 types of foods. Every other food was a "No." I work full-time in retail and am always on my feet, so I had a lot of feet and knee problems. I had constant sinus infections, I was exhausted all the time and I was sick all the time. I had worked with other energy people, but they couldn't get rid of my problems. They could only tell me what my problems were.

With some treatments from Dr. Abel, my pain level decreased from a 7 (on a scale of 1 to 10) to a 2 or 3. I can eat anything now. Abel's treatments have given me my freedom back. Instead of everything being a "No," now everything is a "Yes."

— **Janet Johnson**

When I first went to see Abel, I was feeling terrible. I'd had low back issues since I was a teenager. As an adult, I had abused my body from long hours at work. By the time I got to Abel, I was an absolute mess. Abel's treatments did me so much good, that I have begun learning his style of healing, and am now helping others.

— **Ron Mecchi**

ENERGY
HEALING
UNLOCKED

Discovering the Secrets
of Energy Healing

DR. ABEL RODRIGUEZ

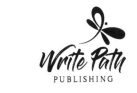

Write Path
PUBLISHING

Kapaa, Kauai, Hawaii 96746
www.WritePath.net

Published by:

PUBLISHING

Kapaa, Hawaii 96746
www.WritePath.net

Cover image: Vivid Graphic Designs / Sky Vreeken
Interior images: Laura Angeli Eliseo
Cover design: Fusion Creative Works
Book interior: Fusion Creative Works
Text font: Minion Pro

Paperback ISBN: 978-0-9970022-0-1
eBook ISBN: 978-0-9970022-3-2
Library of Congress Control Number: 2018956830

This book is dedicated to God for giving me the
answers to my many questions,
and because without God, I would be nothing.

This is also dedicated to Yvette
who inspired me to write this book.

To Shereen

Best Wishes

Axel Rodriguez

Contents

Before we begin

Energy healing works in conjunction with Western medicine, healing energetic blocks to physical healing.

If you have, or suspect you may have a serious medical condition, seek medical help from a licensed physician or other appropriate professional. The energy healing methods contained within this book are meant to compliment traditional medical treatments.

Never stop taking any medication or therapies prescribed by your physician without the direction and supervision of your physician or other health professional. Never advise anyone else to stop taking medication or therapies unless you are their regular physician.

Please do not attempt to help anyone with any physical, emotional or other type of ailment until you are adept at muscle testing, have read this book entirely and have mastered the techniques herein.

Neither the author nor publisher assumes responsibility for improper use of the techniques and/or information contained in this book.

Acknowledgements

I thank my mother for giving me life, strength, a sense of humor, my undying ability to never give up, and for encouraging me to think, think, think.

I thank my father for bringing our family to the United States, and for working diligently to provide for us, in what was a most difficult and scary time for him. He taught me to work hard, to be honest, to do the best I can for other people, and that anything less is a failure.

I thank my childhood best friend, Gary Bachelor, who encouraged me to become a chiropractor. Although he was taken tragically as a young man, he taught me by example to love everybody.

Thanks to my chiropractic teacher, Dr. Dorothea A. Towne, the dean of Cleveland Chiropractic College, for inspiring me to be the best doctor I could be. I always aspired to be at least half as good as she was. Thanks, also, to Dr. Robert Blaich, my first Applied Kinesiology teacher.

My sincere and complete gratitude goes to Dr. George Goodheart, the chiropractor who originated kinesiological muscle testing. Dr. Goodheart's muscle testing led me to discover the methods presented in this book. Without him, many people would still be suffering today, and this book would never have been written.

Thank you to all of my patients throughout the years who unknowingly have been my testing grounds. They have helped me learn, and we have all benefitted.

Thanks go to Yvette, without whose inspiration and support this book probably would never have been written.

Most of all, I thank God for giving me life, my family, my friends and Yvette. God put in my mind and heart the discovery of the methods I share with you in this book. Without God, I would not exist, nor would this book of healing.

Introduction

I suppose it is tempting,
if the only tool you have is a hammer,
to treat everything as if it were a nail.

— Abraham Maslow

Mankind has long been seeking to prevent our most horrible diseases. But we've had only limited success, so we have turned our attention to different ways of treating the thousands and thousands of symptoms that human beings develop.

We try surgery, pharmaceuticals, herbs, vitamins, reflexology, acupuncture, homeopathic remedies, spinal manipulation, faith healing, heat, cold, psychotherapy, physical therapy, sound therapy, color therapy and more. Each of these healing methods is effective in its own way. Yet, millions of people continue to become ill every year.

How could our creator have designed us so perfectly that our heart continues to beat just the right amount at just the right time, with all the intricate functions of our bodies continuing for years, yet we remain susceptible to so many ailments?

Is there something we are failing to see? Are we looking in the wrong place? Are there hints all around us that we don't know how to recognize? What have we been missing?

Maybe the solution is easier than we have ever allowed ourselves to believe.

Throughout this book, I will teach you systems for energy healing. I will show you how to heal in person and how to heal from a distance, from anywhere on the planet. You will learn how to correct the cause of any disorder, and quickly help people heal any condition.

My opinion is that healing comes from a higher source, the life force that is in everything, whether we choose to call it God, Brahma, Allah or the Universe. We are all able to channel this energy for good.

By reading this book, you will learn to harness this energy to help others.

By writing this book, I hope these methods will one day become commonplace.

Dr. Abel Rodriguez

January 2020

ENERGY HEALING

UNLOCKED

Chapter 1
From Hut to Healer

I discovered my Energy Healing Unlocked system inadvertently. Once you know how this unfolded for me, it will be easier to understand and learn my methods for yourself in the chapters that follow. Please take the time to read this first chapter thoroughly, so that subsequent chapters, and the techniques within, make sense to you.

I was born in Veracruz, Mexico, in a small hut with dirt floors. My mother told me that immediately after my birth, my grandmother took me outside our hut, raised me toward the sky and offered my life to God. Until I went to chiropractic college, nothing in my childhood even hinted I would become a healer.

Like most people in Mexico in the 1950s, we were poor. There were few doctors, and we had no money for them anyway. The unschooled local midwife helped deliver me.

My father was an American citizen, born in the United States. At the time of my birth, he was in the U.S. working odd jobs, trying to earn enough money to support our family.

When I was 11 months old, he was able to bring my mother, my older brother, older sister and me to America to start our new life.

Although our family was now together, life was still hard and we were still poor. I remember helping my siblings, parents and grandparents (who had come to California earlier) pick onions in a small town called City of Industry, in Southern California, when I was 2 years old. We pulled the onions from the ground, cut off the tops with tin shears, then placed them into burlap sacks. Sometimes when the foreman felt we were picking onions too slowly, or if we got behind in our quota, he would open up the irrigation ditches. Then we had to pick really fast before the water and mud rushing through the ditches caught up to us. We always lost the race. I have vivid memories of standing and walking in mud, trying to pull heavy bags full of onions through that mud. To this day, if I taste or smell onions, especially combined with the smell of burlap, I become nauseated.

Many days we had nothing to eat. When you are hungry, you will eat practically anything. My mother often sent us to pick weeds in a lot behind our house. She cooked them and told us it was spinach, that it would make us strong like Popeye. The weeds tasted gross, and I never grew muscles like Popeye. As a kid, I thought we must have picked the wrong spinach. We also ate leaves. They tasted like you think they would taste: awful. I did not realize we were poor. I just knew I was hungry.

I can only imagine the heartache and fear my parents must have felt, not being able to feed their children, fearing we would all starve to death. Back then, if you did not have a job or enough money, there was little government aid to help your family with food and shelter. You either worked hard or you went hungry. Few people had abundance, so there were few extras being handed out at the side of the road.

My father began looking for other work. With no experience, he began a gardening business, taking care of people's yards by mowing lawns and pulling weeds. He told me later that he ruined a lot of lawns when he first started, but he soon got the hang of it. When I was about 3 years old, my career changed from onion picker to gardener. My older brother worked with us, too. I know this seems young to be working, but it was a necessity for the children to help with the family business. Hiring employees was expensive, and there was not a lot of yard work business available in those years. By the time I was 5 years old, I was raking leaves and pulling weeds like a pro. But we were still poor and our family was still occasionally eating leaves and weeds.

I usually worked for my father on weekdays after school, on weekends and every day during the summer months. Consequently, I always hated summer. Other kids were ecstatic when the summer began. But me? Not so much.

Childhood Illnesses

I was always a nervous and quiet kid. At the age of 5, I suffered an attack of appendicitis, which led to peritonitis. It felt like I had been punched in the stomach. My father thought I was trying to get out of work by faking an illness — why didn't I think of that? — so he didn't take me to a doctor for a few days. I don't blame him. Health insurance was practically non-existent in the 1950s, and for our family, money for doctors was scarce. Besides, my father was not educated. He did not know about anything more serious than stomach flu.

The doctor told my father to take me to the hospital right away, that my appendix had ruptured and I needed surgery. I had the operation at County General Hospital in Los Angeles, where I spent three weeks recuperating from the surgery as well as from the bacteria and toxins that had escaped into my peritoneum from my ruptured appendix.

At age 7, I developed pneumonia and recovered. When I was 8, I developed tonsillitis. I remember the doctor didn't even look inside my mouth before he told my mother I needed my tonsils removed. He merely gave my mother a price for the operation. The first time he looked down my throat was when he began the actual surgery.

Between illnesses, I continued to work for my father in his gardening business every day after school, on Saturdays, sometimes on Sundays, and all day every day during the summer months. He worked us hard. We often started on people's yards early in the morning, when it was still dark. Our work days ended after it became dark again in the evenings. I remember thinking to myself that a lawnmower with a flashlight attached to it would have really helped.

One of my father's customers was the family whose son was depicted in the movie *Mask,* starring Cher and Sam Elliot. I really felt sorry for the boy. I didn't know at the time what the boy's affliction was, but my heart went out to him. The boy was always so nice. He always asked what I was doing. I always answered, "Raking leaves."

Among the things my father taught me was to always do the best job possible, do it fast, be clean and be honest. These values have stayed with me into adulthood. To this day I still have great respect for manual laborers.

In my teens, I decided that gardening was not in my blood. I didn't know what I was going to do for a living, but I knew I was going to college.

Chiropractic to the Rescue

From his many years of hard manual labor, my father developed severe pain in his lower back. One day at work, he had to crawl to a chain link fence and pull himself up in order to stand. It was really disheartening for me to see my strong father crawl, and it must have been embarrassing for him to know his kids were seeing him in that condition. He finally was able to get home, severely bent over to one side, wracked with pain. I remember feeling scared. Even at my young age, I knew he was our breadwinner. Without him working, we would starve.

The medication prescribed by a physician failed to provide relief, so my father sought out a chiropractor who treated him with spinal adjustments. After only one visit to the chiropractor, my father's pain disappeared and he was able to get back on his feet!

A few years later, my brother injured his back while playing football in school. A physician could do nothing for him, so he was taken to the same chiropractor who treated my father. My brother felt relief, but he needed treatment often to stay out of pain.

As a result of our family's good chiropractic experience, my brother decided to become a chiropractor. When I graduated from high school, I felt God had a destiny for me to do something significant in my life, but I could not put my finger on what it could be. Since my brother and I were close and I looked up to him, I decided to become a chiropractor, too.

After we checked out a few chiropractic schools, we both applied to Cleveland Chiropractic College in Los Angeles, and were both accepted.

Once we started classes and saw the potential health benefits of chiropractic, we felt like we had found the fountain of youth. We were ecstatic.

I graduated from Cleveland Chiropractic College in 1974, and was asked to teach there by the college dean, Dr. Dorothea A. Towne. I had the privilege of teaching at Cleveland for six years, serving as the clinic director for two of those years.

Within a few days of joining the faculty, I realized that I not only loved teaching, I was good at it. I loved reaching into the students' minds and stimulating their senses, their hearts and their intellects. I found I could take the most complex subject and bring it down to an understandable level. I could teach the most boring class by finding ways to show the value of each topic for future use. I continue to love teaching to this day.

My Own Pain

I got married in my early 20s and had two children. The marriage was a disaster. Feeling enormous stress from it, I developed allergies and colds that would last four to six months every year. I began to develop kidney stones, skin diseases, headaches, digestive problems and pain in my lower back. Over time, my back pain became so debilitating that when driving, it felt like my back was on fire. I'd have to stop my car, get out and stand up.

I was still teaching at Cleveland Chiropractic College, so I began to get regular chiropractic spinal adjustments from colleagues, former students and any chiropractors I met during seminars. I probably was adjusted by at least 100 different chiropractors, trying practically every technique known to the profession, but my back pain kept getting worse.

One day in my office, as I bent over to lift a laundry basket of patient gowns, I felt and heard a sharp stabbing "pop" in my low back. The pain was so excruciating that I could not stand up. I felt like I was going to throw up. I couldn't believe this was happening to me.

The pain was so intense, I cancelled all of my appointments for a few days. I went to a few chiropractors seeking relief, but to no avail. Nothing I tried made any difference.

A close friend of mine, Roberto, was a rheumatologist, a physician trained in diseases of the joints, muscles and bones. He gave me a cortisone injection right into my spine. Ouch! He also prescribed anti-inflammatory and pain medication. Finally, after a few days I was able to stand up straight on my own. I thought I was cured.

But as the years passed, my low back pain returned with greater frequency and intensity. My spine became more vulnerable. I became more disabled, and less able to handle almost any physical activity. I found myself protecting my spine as though it was about to break.

I tried eating better and exercising properly, just as I had advised my patients to do. I tried all the spinal exercises prescribed by physicians, chiropractors and physical therapists. In fact, the exercises only exacerbated the pain and increased my disability. I tried massage therapy, acupuncture, reflexology, physical therapy and every other modality known to the chiropractic profession. I got to the point that I could barely walk because of the ever-constant burning pain in my lower back.

I became physically dependent on anti-inflammatory medication, including oral steroids, and painkillers like Darvon and Naprosyn, taking more than the prescribed amounts, yet they only kept the pain down to a level of 8 or 9 on a scale of 0 through 10, with 10 being the worst pain. I could not stand for longer than five seconds without having to sit down, or else I would collapse.

In my own office, I began leaning against a wall while speaking with my patients, so they could not tell I was on the verge of collapse due to pain. I pretended to be relaxed, laid back, no worries.

I did not want my patients to know their chiropractor had back pain that could not be corrected by chiropractic!

Meanwhile, my marriage was falling apart. I tried everything in my power to make it work, but some things are not meant to be. The ongoing stress of trying to save the marriage caused so much pressure on my system that I am amazed I did not have a heart attack. The ensuing divorce broke up my family, caused me to lose my home, my entire savings and the majority of my pension. Life was literally a pain in the back.

Then I met the woman who was to become my second wife. In addition to our wonderful personal life, Yvette managed the day-to-day business of running my practice, scheduling appointments, handling the billing and other office tasks, while I tended to our patients.

But the pain in my lower back remained a nightmare.

One morning I awoke with a sharp gripping pain on one side of my back, and couldn't stand up straight. I told Yvette to have my patients enter the treatment room and lie face down on the treatment table. We told patients their muscles had to relax before the spinal adjustments. After I completed their treatments, I told them to rest on the treatment table a few minutes before getting up, so the spinal adjustments would hold better and longer. The truth was that I did not want patients to see me walk in and out of the treatment room because I was bent over at a 20-degree angle, barely able to stand. My back felt so fragile, like it could break at any moment.

I was in my early 40s by then, and I realized I was heading toward becoming disabled for the rest of my life. I was close to needing a wheelchair. As my pain and disability increased, I became depressed.

Spinal surgery was out of the question for me, as an MRI of my spine revealed I had extensive and severe disc degeneration, which would not respond well to surgery. In all of my years of reading X-rays and MRIs, I had never seen a spine as severely degenerated as mine. I had the spine of a 200-year-old man! How could this have happened to me?

Every night before going to sleep, with tears in my eyes, I prayed to God to heal me. God essentially said, "Not yet." At the time, I could not understand why, but now I understand that God was preparing me for something else.

Enter Applied Kinesiology

In the early years of my chiropractic career, I had heard of a chiropractic specialty technique known as Applied Kinesiology. I heard that it involved some sort of muscle testing, and that it could correct problems that regular spinal adjustments could not. Now, in my desperation to solve my own seemingly unsolvable back pain, I decided to find a chiropractor who used this technique.

I searched the city where I lived and surrounding communities, but could find no one who had the experience I needed. Again, I prayed to God asking for help, and I waited, and I suffered.

Then, one day out of the blue, I got a postcard from a chiropractor who was teaching Applied Kinesiology in Los Angeles. Out of desperation, I decided to take the course. Maybe it could help.

I was immediately impressed with the instructor's knowledge of muscles and body systems. As I watched demonstrations during this course, I saw the technique required a lot of study and practice. This was why so few chiropractors used Applied Kinesiology — or were good at it.

The course instructor, Robert Blaich, D.C., lived and practiced in Denver, Colorado. I began traveling from California to Denver for treatment with him. I noticed only slight improvements at first, but I had great confidence in Dr. Blaich's treatments, so I flew to Denver twice a month. I saw him for three hours on Monday mornings, three hours Monday afternoons, did the same on Tuesdays, then flew home on Tuesday nights. Back in my own office on Wednesday morning, I attempted to treat my patients.

After about six months of treatment with Dr. Blaich, my back pain finally began to subside and my mobility improved. On a 0-to-10 scale, my pain reduced from 8 or 9 down to 2 or 3. I decreased my treatment frequency with Dr. Blaich to once a month, then down to three times per year.

Retirement . . . Or Not

I was feeling so much better that I decided not to push my luck. So after four years of treatment with Dr. Blaich I retired to the Hawaiian island of Kauai, something I had dreamed of doing for many years.

On Kauai, it was a pleasure for me to be able to exercise without pain. I was also able to sit quietly and have time to smell the hibiscus, so to speak. (A hibiscus doesn't have much fragrance, but you get the idea.) For the first time in 48 years — my whole life — I was able to kick back and do absolutely nothing, just relax.

But after many days at the beach, drinking mai tais and piña coladas, I felt I was not being useful. I began giving free chiropractic treatments to members of our church. I didn't realize yet that God was pulling on my heartstrings.

Soon I began to run across people who complained of spinal pain and other health problems. I recommended they find a practicing chiropractor. Many people said they had done so, but the treatments had not helped them, or their pain got worse. I could probably have helped them, but I was not in practice.

One day, as I was driving home from the grocery store, I heard a strong spiritual voice ask me, "What have you done for my children?" Somehow, I knew the question came from God. Until that moment, I had always believed that people who thought God was talking to them were really just talking to themselves. But the message I received was overwhelming and would not go away. I realized that when I die, I will have to stand before God and answer his question, "What have you done for my children?" I could have been helping God's children more than I had, instead of concerning myself only with my own comfort.

When I got home, I told my wife about my message from God and that I was ready to go back into practice.

When I opened my office on Kauai, I decided to use Applied Kinesiology and muscle testing. They are the foundation for my method of unlocking energy healing, and I will teach you about them in the following chapters.

Curing Gluten Intolerance

When I first began to study and practice Applied Kinesiology, I kept thinking there must be a better way than simply telling people they had to avoid something they liked eating or doing for the rest of their lives. I trusted my doubts, and was led on a gradual unfoldment of the mysteries that had puzzled me.

My path of discovery began with a bad cold. I had always been susceptible to severe colds that lasted three to four months and occurred two or three times a year. One day, while suffering one of my usual long, miserable colds, I felt like an overinflated balloon, ready to burst. I took my own blood pressure. The systolic pressure was 205. Normal is around 120. I panicked!

I cancelled my patient appointments and raced to the emergency room. A physician saw my laboratory work and put me on high blood pressure medication. He said I probably would have to be on high blood pressure medicine for the rest of my life.

I did not want to face a lifetime of dealing with side effects and other health problems from blood pressure medications, so I contacted an applied kinesiologist chiropractor whose DVDs I had studied from, and flew to see him in Nevada. After my second visit, my blood pressure was under control. (I had — and still have — tremendous respect and gratitude for Dr. Blaich, the chiropractor in Denver who helped my back pain heal. I called a different chiropractor this time only to find out if I could learn something more about Applied Kinesiology.)

As I was getting ready to leave his office, the Nevada chiropractor said something that changed my life. "You know you are gluten intolerant, right?"

I did know. Dr. Blaich had told me years before, explaining that my body did not digest regular wheat flour used to make bread, cookies, pasta, cakes, pies and other types of food. He told me that gluten intolerance was one of the reasons for my back pain and inflammation, and that I needed to eliminate all forms of flour from my diet for the rest of my life. This depressed me. What the heck was I going to do without any baked goods for the rest of my life?

From Dr. Blaich I had learned gluten intolerance was a huge problem associated with hundreds of symptoms and conditions such as diabetes, irritable bowel syndrome, allergies, high blood pressure, high cholesterol, and some say autism and even cancer. I learned wheat flour is used in many foods, and as a thickening agent in many soups and sauces, like tomato soup. Wheat flour is used in many desserts and also in beer. Wheat flour is even part of the spice mixture in the corn chip Doritos. Wheat is everywhere.

When Dr. Blaich explained to me that I was gluten intolerant, I realized life as I knew it was over. But I was willing to do whatever it took to get well. If going gluten-free was the price I had to pay to live pain-free, I was willing to pay it. What choice did I have? I could stay in a wheelchair and eat all the gluten I wanted, or I could quit eating gluten foods and live without pain, able to walk again with ease.

So I had not eaten gluten for seven years. Now, talking with the chiropractor in Nevada, I asked if he could correct the problem. "No, it can't be fixed," he replied. "Nobody can fix it." He explained that all humans are born without the enzyme to break down gluten, that gluten was never meant for humans and was meant only for animals. He said that thousands of years ago Egyptians incorporated gluten into their diet and passed the habit to the rest of humanity. "That's why we have all the problems with gluten intolerance today," he told me.

Thank God he said this to me. He made me question the accepted "facts" about gluten.

On my flight home to Kauai, I was feeling sorry for myself. While I had not gone to see him for gluten intolerance, I had hoped one day to find someone who could desensitize my body so I could eat foods containing flour again. He dashed that hope.

Then I thought to myself, "Wait a minute. *This just doesn't make sense.* If all humans are born without the enzyme to break down the gluten in wheat flour, then *nobody* should be able to eat gluten. Why can millions of people eat wheat flour with no trouble, while millions of us are so intolerant or allergic that eating any wheat flour can be life threatening?"

The more I thought about it during the flight, the more I knew some sort of organ dysfunction had to be causing gluten intolerance. So why not cure the cause?

When I arrived home, I excitedly told Yvette about my new reasoning: If gluten intolerance is caused by some part of the body not functioning properly, then there had to be some way to correct the dysfunction and the intolerance using Applied Kinesiology techniques.

My wife, who had been with me every step of the way, watching me suffer from debilitating back pain, then helping me avoid gluten, was scared. She was unwilling to see me immobilized again. Since Yvette stood by me through everything in my personal life, including my decision to come out of retirement, bringing her out of retirement with me, I gave her veto power in areas I wanted her support.

"Abel, you are not going to eat flour," she said. "So forget about it."

"What if I can cure it?"

"You are *not* eating flour. The answer is no."

"What if I *prove* that I have cured it?"

"You are not having flour."

"What if I cure it to your satisfaction?"

Her eyes widened. "To my satisfaction?"

"Yes, to your satisfaction."

"Yes, if you do that, then you can have flour again."

"Yes" is such a beautiful word.

Within minutes of Yvette saying "Yes," I began praying to God, asking for proof humans are meant to eat gluten. In a few seconds I received a vision of Jesus giving bread to the apostles at the Last Supper (Matthew 26:26). Who would know better than Jesus if flour wasn't meant for us? The thought convinced me beyond doubt. I decided the belief we humans do not have the enzymes to break down gluten must be mistaken.

Now I had to find a way to correct the intolerance that we humans have somehow inadvertently created. I knew in my heart it could be done. Again, I prayed to God to show me how to do it. Within a few minutes, an answer came to me.

According to Applied Kinesiology, if a person is gluten intolerant, tasting flour or holding flour to the abdomen will weaken a person's muscles, as evidenced during muscle testing, a technique I will teach you in Chapter 2.

The next day, my first patient happened to be gluten intolerant. I proceeded to do the treatment I had envisioned the night before, that took only minutes. (You'll learn actual treatments, or "corrections," as I call them, in Chapter 6.)

At the end of the session, I told the patient to go home and eat one bite of bread. If there was no negative reaction by the next day, he could eat a little more bread, and again check for any reaction. He could slowly increase his bread intake as long as his body was tolerating the gluten. I told him to stop eating gluten if there were *any* negative symptoms. His body indicated a correction for gluten intolerance had been made, I said, but his body would need time to fully correct itself.

A week later, the patient returned to my office for a follow-up visit. He began the session by thanking me profusely. He said he had been eating bread, pizza, spaghetti and cookies all week. In fact, he was eating all the bread and pasta he could get his hands on.

"No, wait!" I said, "You were supposed to eat only a little bread at a time, so you integrated gluten back into your diet slowly."

"I know," he replied, "but once I realized that I no longer got sick from eating gluten, well, I couldn't stop myself."

I was shocked, but I did not let on that he was the first person on whom I'd tried my new technique. Inside I thought, "This might work on one in a thousand people, and I got him right away."

Later that day, I tried the technique on another patient with gluten intolerance. I gave the same instruction to go slowly. This patient began eating wheat right away, and had no negative reactions. "Okay," I thought, "two in a thousand."

I tried the procedure on the next patient who came to my office with gluten intolerance. After the treatment, she also was able to eat flour immediately without getting sick. Apparently I was onto something.

I kept correcting gluten intolerance in patient after patient. Some ate gluten foods right after they left the office and had no negative effects. Some had to return for corrections two or three times, but more than 90 percent of my patients required only one treatment.

They could eat all of the wheat-based foods they wanted, often the same day, with no signs of intolerance.

The correction for gluten intolerance was immediate, and seemed to be permanent.

Naturally, I soon addressed my own gluten intolerance. After I did the correction, Yvette muscle tested me. Once she was satisfied I had, indeed, corrected the gluten intolerance in myself, she let me eat a bite of bread.

I did not have any negative reaction. Such a happy day in my life! I began eating gluten foods like cookies, pies, pasta and lots of bread. I have not had a single flare-up of low back pain since 2007, when that correction was done. I had cured my gluten intolerance once and for all!

Taking it to the Next Step

A few months later, I asked myself, "If this technique corrects gluten intolerance, will it correct intolerances to lactose, corn, oats, peanuts, tomatoes, coffee, shellfish and other foods?" I tested this with patients who had these intolerances. To my amazement, they all corrected with *no* exceptions. I thought I was dreaming. How could I have discovered a way to correct food intolerances so easily? Why had no one else been teaching this procedure?

I realized that for some people, these intolerances were allergies, such as an allergy to bee stings. I began using my technique to correct allergies of all types. Again to my astonishment, all the allergies I corrected soon disappeared. I started correcting allergies to cats, dogs, pollens, dust, mold, grass, poison oak, poison ivy and so on. The results continued to amaze me. How far could this new procedure be extended?

One day a new patient, Jason F., came into my office because his friends told him about me doing "miraculous cures." He asked if I could cure diabetes. Humbled, I explained to him that I had no special power to cure him or anyone. I could help his body cure itself by removing whatever his body revealed through Applied Kinesiology and muscle testing to be the *cause* of his diabetes.

I had never treated diabetes before, but I thought if I could localize and correct the cause, in theory, his body would be able to reverse the permanent shut down and atrophy of the pancreas.

Jason said, "If you're willing to try, I am, too."

Using Applied Kinesiology to guide my corrections, I treated what we identified as the cause of his diabetes. Within a few treatments, his blood sugar and insulin returned to normal levels. His physician eventually told him he could stop taking insulin. I was startled. My simple procedure had produced a dramatic life-changing reversal of an organ's disease process. Something was happening that I did not yet understand.

New Dimension

As I kept learning and developing my new technique, I started correcting jaw problems, headaches, knee pains, digestive and hormonal disturbances, and other ailments. With only a few minutes of treatment, most conditions were corrected, and the majority required only one treatment.

When one of my patients brought in her sister, Linda, who was diagnosed with severe schizophrenia and multiple personality disorder, a new dimension opened in my practice.

Linda could barely remember her kids and could barely respond to my questions. While taking her case history, I asked her, "Do you know you are schizophrenic?"

She did not answer.

I asked, "Do you know if there is somebody else living inside of you, speaking to you?"

She did not respond. Something told me to persist. Somehow I knew I was on the right track.

I again asked, "Is there someone else inside of you?"

Finally, she raised her head slightly. From her prescription drug-induced stupor, she nodded and whispered, "Yes."

I decided to approach her mental disorder like any other dysfunction in any other patient. I would leave it up to God. If God wanted to use me to help her get well, then God would have to put in my mind a way to help this poor woman.

I started to work on identifying and correcting the *cause* of Linda's mental illness, which had its roots in her emotions. She first came to my office on a Monday. By Thursday of that week, she entered the office with a great big smile on her face. She was a completely different person, laughing with me and speaking normally. She said that she felt normal for the first time in years. Her sister confirmed she had not seen Linda this way in a long time.

Soon after treating Linda, I was flooded with patients asking me to correct depression, obsessive-compulsive disorder, bipolar syndrome, phobias, dyslexia, ADD/ADHD, autism, addiction and many other mental and emotional disorders. Working with these patients helped me figure out how to find the source of every mental and emotional disorder. I was learning to cure any ailment by correcting the cause.

I kept expanding the scope of conditions I could treat successfully, such as arthritis, migraine headaches, hormonal imbalances, digestive disturbances, skin diseases, high blood pressure, high cholesterol, cardiovascular disease, knee problems, tumors, plantar fasciitis and respiratory diseases.

Yvette and I moved back to the mainland from Hawaii and opened an office in California. Word spread about all the different physical and mental conditions I could successfully correct. I became busier than ever.

Emotions: The Root Cause

At the time I was learning to correct these diseases and disorders, my sole purpose was to improve my treatment techniques, and to help my patients get well faster, with fewer visits.

I had no idea that I was slowly meandering through a maze that would lead me to the root cause of disease.

I became more sophisticated in my technique and began to discover that numerous pains and diseases were not being caused by abnormal reflexes or organ dysfunctions, but about 50 percent of the time by emotions.

For example, an allergy could be caused by a dysfunctioning small intestine in one patient, which in turn had its roots in emotions. In another patient, an allergy could be caused by emotions directly.

I am not the first person in the world to discover the power of emotions. However, until that time I had never learned this in any of my courses of study, nor experience. God was leading me on this path for a reason.

Soon I began muscle testing for emotions *first* as the primary cause of my patients' various ailments. When muscle testing indicated that emotions were not directly responsible, I returned to testing organs or musculoskeletal parts, as I had always done.

Gradually, the percentage of time my muscle testing indicated emotions as the primary cause began rising from 50 percent to 60, then to 70, until finally it reached 100 percent of the time. My patients' bodies no longer signaled that organs or musculoskeletal structures were the actual cause of anything. Every patient's body indicated that emotions were the root cause. (I will detail this in Chapter 4.)

Distance Healing

One day I wondered, "Can we heal any patient with thoughts projected from a distance?"

I tried an experiment. While in the same room as the people I was trying to treat, I stood a few feet away from them as I did my procedures. I also tested this method with friends and family members who were hundreds of miles away. Much to my astonishment, the healing processes took place.

I realized that *energy healing is not bound by time or space.* I launched more experiments. I attempted to treat patients thousands of miles away, and *it worked!* I could heal patients across great distances with results as good as with patients in the same room.

Refining my discovery, I began treating patients over the telephone. Everything I was trying to correct for them actually corrected. The treatments worked as fast and as effectively as if they were in my treatment room.

Ready to Do it Yourself?

Now that you know the story of how I became an energy healer, are you ready to learn how to do it yourself? The rest of this book is devoted to teaching you the code for energy healing.

I will show you how to heal in person and how to heal from a distance. We will move step-by-step through the techniques. Some of the methods will come easily to you. Some may not. I suggest asking a friend or spouse to be your practice partner. The more you use these techniques, the more adept you will become.

Think of what you are about to learn as if it is the code to a push-button lock on a door. If you push buttons randomly without knowing the code, you cannot open the door. Once you learn the correct code, you will be able to unlock all doors easily, through energy healing.

> *Everyone has the gift of energy healing,*
> *but it takes time and practice.*

After reading this book, and with practice at muscle testing and clear-thinking, you will learn how to correct the cause of any disorder and quickly help people heal any condition.

My opinion is that healing comes from a higher power, the life force that is in everything, whether we choose to call it God, Brahma, Allah or the Universe. We are all able to channel this energy for good.

Whatever you wish to call it, you will learn to harness this energy to help others. Practice diligently, have patience with yourself and prepare to be amazed.

Chapter 2
Muscle Testing

"Know what *you are thinking and* how *you are thinking."*
— *Dr. Abel Rodriguez*

Kinesiology is the study of movement and motion, such as how a bullet flies through the air, how a leaf falls to the ground, how a truck travels down a road or how electrons move around a nucleus. The study of human motion and movement, the action of one muscle, or groups of muscles influencing another muscle or groups of muscles, is human kinesiology.

Applied Kinesiology is a system in which practitioners "muscle test," causing muscles to either weaken or strengthen. Applied Kinesiology practitioners believe muscle testing is the best way to isolate what is causing physical dysfunction, and to determine how to help.

While I am not going to teach you how to become an applied kinesiologist, I will teach you how to muscle test in order to perform the majority of the techniques in this book.

Muscle Testing Basics

The most important concept to understand is that muscle testing in Applied Kinesiology is **not** based on conventional strength. Even a bodybuilder's muscle will weaken if you are testing a substance that is harmful to him, or testing an organ in his body that is not functioning properly. (Note: I say "him" for simplicity. Every concept in this book applies equally to persons of any gender.)

For example, if my patient touches his liver reflex while I muscle test, his strong muscle will weaken if the liver reflex is dysfunctioning. This is the body's way of telling us there is something wrong with the liver reflex and possibly the liver itself.

(Reflex points are places on the body that, when touched, cause organs or muscles to have a reflex action. For the purposes of this book, that's all you need to understand about reflex points.)

The concept of muscle testing is that you are looking for a change in the strength of the muscle you are testing. When a strong muscle weakens or a weak muscle strengthens, you have received an answer from the body. This change in muscle strength is telling you that whatever you are testing is either harmful or beneficial to the body.

*It is the change in muscle response
from strong to weak,
or from weak to strong,
that you are looking for.*

The beauty and power of muscle testing is that you are able to zero in on exactly what is causing issues in each patient's body. As one of my patients says, "I want my treatment to be based on *my* body, not someone else's."

Why Does Muscle Testing Work?

Muscle testing works because the body is responding to your inquiries by either allowing or disallowing energy flow. Some patients report that it feels like their arm is powered by an infinite source when their muscle tests strong. When it tests weak, the power is temporarily disconnected from its source. Your results should be this consistent, regardless of your patient's actual physical strength.

Muscle testing is an amazing tool, the magnitude of which is, at first, beyond most people's imagination. We can ask our bodies about anything that is not working properly, and how to correct it. Inquiries to the body can be about topics ranging from reflex points, to structures (bones, ligaments, tendons, muscles), sutures (where two bones in the skull come together), or emotions, as you will learn.

There are no side effects to muscle testing when done correctly.

Therapy Localization

Before you learn how to muscle test, you'll need to understand the concept of Therapy Localization, a method that applied kinesiologists have used for decades in conjunction with muscle testing.

The principle of Therapy Localization, as typically taught, is that if a patient touches a part or organ reflex on their body and there is some kind of dysfunction with that part, this will cause a strong muscle in their body to weaken, indicating that there is something wrong with that body part.

Conversely if a patient has a weak muscle and they touch a part or organ reflex on their body that is causing or contributing to that muscle being weak, this will cause that previously weak muscle to become strong.

Muscle testing in this manner pinpoints where to localize the therapy. It tells the tester where to provide treatment.

In using the theory of Therapy Localization, you place a food item or other substance on the abdomen or tongue of a patient, then muscle test. The concept is that if the muscle weakens, the patient is intolerant to that substance, and/or the substance is causing some sort of harm to the body. For the purposes of this book, intolerance encompasses hearing, seeing, smelling, touching, tasting or even simply thinking of something or someone that causes emotional or physical upset.

For example, it is very common for practitioners to place a small container of wheat flour (gluten) on a patient's abdomen, then muscle test. When the patient's muscle weakens during testing, the patient is told they are gluten intolerant.

Conversely if you place a substance on someone's tongue or on their body that is beneficial for them, such as a vitamin, it will strengthen every weak muscle in their body.

However, in my experience with thousands patients and counting, neither the presence of the food item, nor the touching of any particular body part, causes the muscle to weaken while testing.

It is the question or statement you are asking the body that creates the muscle weakening or strengthening.

For example, when a skilled applied kinesiologist places a small container of wheat flour on a patient's abdomen and begins muscle testing, the applied kinesiologist will be thinking "the concept of Joe being gluten intolerant." The practitioner may not consciously realize they have asked a question, however, the intent behind placing the flour on the patient's stomach and muscle testing is indeed asking the question.

The body responds to this, producing the patient's muscle weakening, if the patient is gluten intolerant. The bag of wheat flour is merely a prop to keep the mind focused. Once you can hold laser-like focus in your mind on the topics for which you are muscle testing, you will no longer need the visual aids.

This distinction is of critical importance. When you are testing tangible items, such as wheat flour or sugar, it is fine to use visual aids. But you need a method for testing intangible things, such as when working with diseases or mental issues.

That's why my motto is: **Know *what* you are thinking and *how* you are thinking.** When you understand this concept, you are on your way to unlocking the true power of energy healing.

Your Thoughts Direct the Energy

For those of you familiar with muscle testing, it may be new to you that it is the question or statement you are asking the body that creates the muscle weakening or strengthening, rather than the simple presence of the harmful or beneficial item. Our intent, or expectation, tells the body to let us know, via muscle testing, whether a substance is beneficial or harmful. I will teach you how to test this for yourself at the end of the chapter.

Your thoughts direct the flow of energy.

This may be the opposite of what you previously learned about muscle testing. The reality is all of us have more power to heal each other than we, as a human race, have believed for centuries.

Muscle Testing Mechanics

Note #1: I use the word "patient" in this book to represent the person on whom you are learning muscle testing techniques, i.e. your practice subject. Please do ***not*** attempt to help anyone with any physical, emotional or other any type of ailment until you are adept at muscle testing and you have read this book entirely.

Note #2: While you are learning muscle testing, it is paramount to practice on someone who is relatively healthy. Even though muscle testing is not a function of physical strength, it can be taxing on people who have significant health issues.

Now, let's learn how to muscle test!

Muscle testing can be done with practically any muscle in the body. My preference for repeated testing is a shoulder muscle called the pectoralis major (clavicular division), which runs from the clavicle or collarbone to the top of the humerus, the bone in the upper arm. (Refer to image.) I have found this muscle is weak on most people on their right side, so I recommend using the left side.

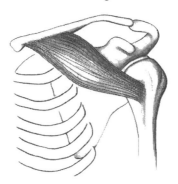

Pectoralis major muscle

I prefer this muscle because other muscles typically weaken after about half a dozen tests, while the pectoralis muscle seems to be able to test indefinitely.

Ask your "patient" to lie down on his or her back on a table (massage or chiropractic tables are most comfortable), or on a bench. Sit or stand at the middle of the head of the table. Ask the patient to raise his or her left arm so it is perpendicular to their body, with the palm of their hand facing at a 45-degree angle away from the body.

Place your right hand gently on the patient's right shoulder to keep them from rolling to left or right.

Then, as you tell the patient to "Resist," lightly push against the outside of their forearm, near the wrist, along that same 45-degree angle. Sometimes I will say "Pull" and tell patients to aim for my face so they understand which direction to pull their arm, as some are confused the first time. (Refer to images.)

The patient's muscle will either immediately lock, or you will easily be able to push their arm down an inch or so.

If the muscle weakens and does not lock, stop pushing. Do not, under any circumstance, push the arm all the way down.

The maximum amount of pressure you should use will vary from patient to patient, however it should never cause pain or discomfort to the patient.

If muscle testing causes any discomfort in your patient, stop immediately.

It will take practice to feel the initial lock of a muscle, and to discern when a muscle is not going to lock. That's why it's imperative to practice on relatively healthy people whose muscles don't tire easily.

***M**uscle testing is not a contest of strength. You are looking only for the muscle to lock, to stay in place while gently pushing the forearm near the wrist, feeling only for the first phase of resistance, which will take place immediately, if the muscle is going to lock at all.*

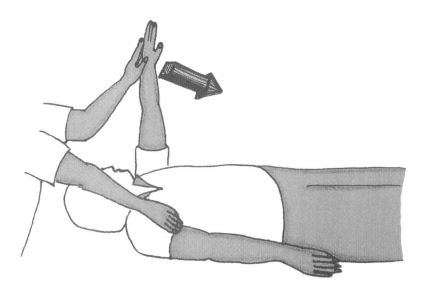

Muscle testing using the pectoralis major (clavicular division), which runs from the clavicle or collarbone to the top of the humerus, the bone in the upper arm. I recommend using the left side. Have the patient raise his or her left arm so it is perpendicular to the floor, with the palm of their hand facing at 45-degree angle away from the body. As you tell the patient to "Resist," lightly push against the outside of their forearm, near the wrist, along that same 45-degree angle.

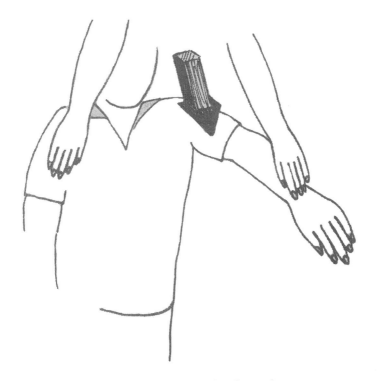

Muscle testing, overhead view.

Alternate Testing Muscles

At times you will need to use a different muscle for testing, such as if the patient has a rotator cuff injury, rheumatoid arthritis or other significant injury or disease affecting the shoulder area, or if the left pectoralis major muscle won't test strong before you begin your diagnostics.

First, try the right pectoralis major muscle, though, as mentioned earlier, the right side often tests weak in most people.

You can test with the quadriceps or the tensor fascia lata muscles, both located in the thigh. If your patient can only be tested using these muscles, I recommend you learn on someone else, as these muscles tend to exhaust very quickly.

Testing with Quadriceps Muscle

To test using the quadriceps muscle, begin with your patient lying on his or her back with one knee bent at approximately a 90-degree angle. Place your hand on the thigh, two to three inches above the kneecap of the bent leg and push toward the feet. (Refer to image.) Tell them to resist your push, to pull their knee toward their shoulder. If the patient's quadriceps can test strong, the muscle will lock in place. Note: the quadriceps muscle tests weak in many people.

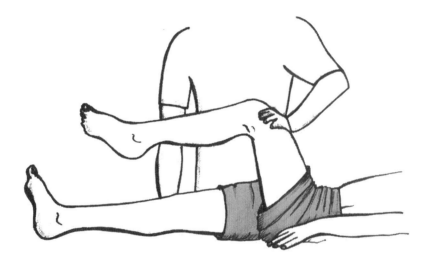

An alternate for muscle testing is the quadriceps muscle. Patient lies on his or her back with one knee bent at a 90-degree angle. Place your hand on the thigh, two to three inches above the kneecap of the bent leg and push toward the feet, while the patient resists.

Testing with Tensor Fascia Lata Muscle

To test using the tensor fascia lata muscle, have the person lie on his or her back, raising one of their legs one to two feet off the table, diagonally to the side about 15 to 20 degrees, and rotated inward, also approximately 15 to 20 degrees. Their knee should be completely extended (not bent). Place your hand on the outside of their ankle and push diagonally down toward the table, toward their other leg. Have them resist by pushing their leg outward. (Refer to image.) Note: the tensor fascia lata muscle tests weak in many people.

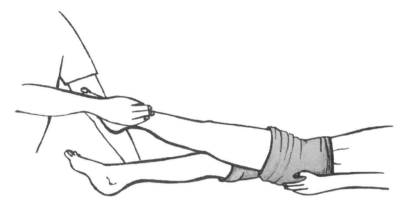

To test using the tensor fascia lata muscle, have the person raise one of their legs one to two feet off the table, diagonally to the side about 15 to 20 degrees, rotated inward, also approximately 15 to 20 degrees. Their knee should be completely extended (not bent). Place your hand on the outside of their ankle and push diagonally down toward the table, toward their other leg, while the patient resists.

No matter which muscle you choose to test, remember this is **not** a contest of strength. You are looking only for the muscle to immediately lock, to stay in place while gently pushing. Likewise, your patient will not need to exert much pressure for their muscle to lock, if it is going to lock at all.

Getting Started

The first thing you need to decide is how the body will indicate to you whether something is harmful or beneficial to your patient. You do this by setting your intent.

You have four options, below, though you only need the first two to learn my Energy Healing Unlocked system:

1. On a YES answer, a strong muscle will become weak if you intend it to become weak.
2. On a NO answer, a strong muscle will remain strong if you intend it to remain strong.
3. On a YES answer, a weak muscle will become strong if you intend it to become strong.
4. On a NO answer, a weak muscle will remain weak if you intend it to remain weak.

Begin with a strong muscle, then expect, or tell, the body to weaken that muscle, as a way of signaling if a statement is true.

To determine if the muscle you want to use is "strong," begin testing the patient's left pectoralis major muscle, as described earlier, with their free hand lying at their side. If the muscle locks immediately with slight pressure, it is strong.

If the muscle won't lock, first try retesting with less pressure, as you may be pushing too hard. Remember, muscle testing requires only a minimum of pressure, and pushing the arm down one inch maximum. If the muscle still won't lock, try testing alternate muscles as described earlier.

Once you find a strong muscle, you are ready to begin asking questions.

Say out loud something like this: "The concept of a dysfunction of the liver reflex," while the person being tested touches their liver reflex with their free hand. Speaking aloud aligns your mind with the body part being tested.

Next, tell the person to "Resist," as you gently push their arm down in the 45-degree angle I have described. If there is a liver dysfunction, the muscle will immediately weaken.

(See illustration of chart of reflexes. As I mentioned earlier, reflex points are places on the body that, when touched, cause organs or muscles to have a reflex action. For the purposes of this book, that's all you need to understand about reflex points.)

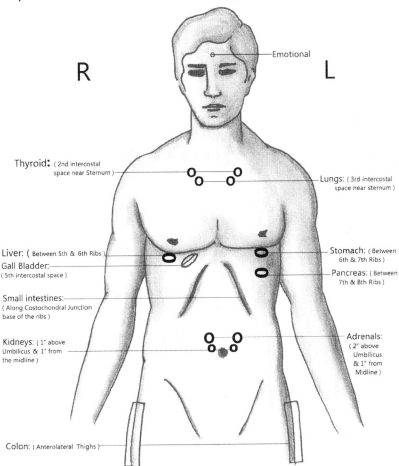

R   Emotional   L

Thyroid: (2nd intercostal space near Sternum)

Lungs: (3rd intercostal space near sternum)

Liver: (Between 5th & 6th Ribs)
Gall Bladder:
(5th intercostal space)

Stomach: (Between 6th & 7th Ribs)

Pancreas: (Between 7th & 8th Ribs)

Small intestines:
(Along Costochondral Junction base of the ribs)

Kidneys: (1" above Umbilicus & 1" from the midline)

Adrenals:
(2" above Umbilicus & 1" from Midline)

Colon: (Anterolateral Thighs)

Basic chart of reflexes. Reflex points are places on the body that, when touched, cause organs or muscles to have a reflex action. For the purposes of this book, that's all you need to understand about reflex points.

Resetting the Muscle to Strong

Any time you receive an answer in the form a weak muscle, "reset" the muscle to strong before continuing.

Do this by clearing your mind of questions, then telling the patient to "resist" while lightly pushing against the outside of their forearm (assuming you are testing with their pectoralis major).

When you feel the lock again, the muscle has tested strong and is ready for more questions.

Crystal Clear

The body can only answer you by signaling "Yes" or "No," so reliable muscle testing depends on you being crystal clear about what you are thinking. Additionally, you must ask only one question or statement per muscle test, because the body can answer only one question at a time.

For example, if you are testing how sugar affects your patient, make the statement: "This person is intolerant to sugar." If the person is intolerant to sugar, the muscle will weaken. The body is telling you that your statement is correct. However, if the muscle stays strong, the body is telling you that your statement is incorrect.

By contrast, if you think about sugar in general, without asking if your specific patient is intolerant to it, the muscle won't weaken because you have not asked the question clearly enough. The body lacks a way of replying, "Yes, it is sugar, and what about it?"

Keep practicing until you get good at having complete focus and clarity in your mind while testing.

Second Nature

Muscle testing sounds simple — and it is — but you must practice to become good at it. You may need anywhere from a few minutes to a few weeks to get a feeling for how to do it correctly and accurately.

Practice until it becomes second nature to you. Reach the point where you can sense a muscle locking with a minimum of thought. Reach the point where you are barely thinking about the arm or muscle testing itself, but rather about the substance, body part or ailment you are asking about.

Muscle testing must become as natural to you as breathing.

Feel free to use items as visual aids while learning to keep your focus, such as wheat flour, sugar or whatever food items you want to test, until you no longer need them.

Take as much time as you need to learn. Don't give up! You *will* get it. Remember, there are no accidents. You are reading this book for a reason.

Muscle Testing Tips & Pointers

Begin with a Strong Muscle — If a person's muscle doesn't test strong from the outset, try their quadriceps or tensor fascia lata muscles as described earlier in this chapter. If those muscles don't test strong, find a different person to practice on.

Reset the Muscle — Any time you receive an answer in the form a weak muscle, "reset" the muscle to strong before continuing. Do this by clearing your mind of questions, then telling the patient to "resist" while lightly pushing against the muscle you have chosen to test. When the muscle locks, proceed with your next question.

Clear, Open Mind — Keep your mind clear and open. Any bias or insertion of your own opinion will give inaccurate results. Remember, this process is not about what you think is happening in the patient's body. It is about what each patient's body is telling you.

Test a Variety — While you are developing your muscle testing skills, begin testing with easy questions that you know the answer to, such as "This person's name is John" or "We are in the state of California."

Graduate to testing a variety of things related to bodily functions and health to learn how it feels when a muscle tests weak.

For example, test your "patient's" liver reflex. If the muscle tests strong, it is possible that person's liver reflex is functioning normally. Move onto their other reflexes. You are bound to find something that is not functioning at optimum levels, as is the case with most humans.

Trust — Trust that muscle testing works, and don't over-think the mechanics. It's similar to learning how to swim. If you kick your feet and stroke your arms, you will, indeed, swim. Like most anything, the more you do it, the more natural it feels.

Graduate Level 1

Once you become proficient at muscle testing, prove to yourself that it is not the mere presence of a harmful or beneficial item that causes a muscle to weaken or strengthen, but rather, your focus.

Have your "patient" touch an organ reflex, let's say the liver reflex. The liver reflex is a safe bet as most people's livers are not functioning at their optimum level. Muscle test, and if there is anything wrong with the liver, the muscle will weaken. (If the muscle remains strong while testing the liver reflex, choose a different organ reflex, such as the stomach reflex.) For the purposes of this exercise, let's assume the liver reflex weakened the muscle.

Reset the muscle to strong. Now, have the patient continue touching their liver reflex — only this time, think of sitting on a sunny beach near the ocean, skiing on a mountain or strolling alongside a river. Muscle test again. The muscle will remain strong, because your focus has shifted away from the patient's liver.

Your focus directs the energy.

Graduate Level 2

Once you become adept at muscle testing, you no longer will need to speak your questions or statements out loud to keep your mind focused. You will be able to merely think them and the muscle will respond correctly.

Have your "patient" touch their liver reflex and muscle test. For the purposes of this example, let's assume that the muscle weakens. (If it doesn't weaken, test organ reflexes until you find one that does.)

Reset the muscle to strong. Now, have the patient stop touching their liver reflex, returning their arm to their side. Simply *visualize* the patient touching their liver reflex, and muscle test. The muscle will weaken as if the patient was actually touching their liver reflex.

Energy follows your focus.

Developing your focus so that it becomes this laser sharp will be a major step toward unlocking your ability to do energy healing in seconds rather than weeks, months or years. Initially, this might not seem like much of a time savings from saying things aloud, but it will be when you begin to fire questions at the body at lightning speed, helping heal more complex ailments or those that have causes that are not obvious.

Graduate Level 3

Once you become an expert at both muscle testing and holding your focus on where the body is leading you, you can speed up your testing. Instead of resetting the muscle to strong after each time a response weakens it, you can instead note the *change* in muscle response from weak to strong, or strong to weak. To do this, set this as your intention before a round of testing.

It can take some time to understand where the body is leading you via alternating strengths of the muscle, so for the purposes of this book, we will always reset the muscle to strong after each time it weakens.

≈ ≈ ≈

Let's pause here to grasp the enormity of the tool of muscle testing. Do you see the magnificence of this? We can use muscle testing to tell us practically everything we want to know about a patient's body.

It is my belief that the body is simply the medium or messenger for God or Universal wisdom. The body must have an IQ of 50 trillion to the trillionth power!

Once we accept that *pure energy* allows muscles to respond, the world opens up to us — if we use the tool wisely. We only need to know what to ask and how to ask it. This is Energy Healing Unlocked.

CAUTION: Please feel free to continue reading this book while you are establishing your muscle testing techniques. However, I recommend refraining from attempting healing work until you become proficient at muscle testing.

Muscle Testing
Chapter Summary

1. Kinesiology is the study of motion and movement, including the action of one muscle, or groups of muscles influencing another muscle or groups of muscles.

2. Applied kinesiologists frequently apply a technique called "muscle testing" to diagnose what is ailing a patient and determine how best to help.

3. The concept of muscle testing is that you are looking for a change in the strength of the muscle you are testing. When a strong muscle weakens, or a weak muscle strengthens, you have received an answer from the body.

4. Muscle testing is *not* a contest of physical strength. Muscle testing works because the body responds to your inquiries by either allowing or disallowing energy flow.

5. Therapy Localization is a diagnostic procedure in which body parts or external items are muscle tested to determine if there is an imbalance or dysfunction in the body, and/or if certain substances are helping or harming the body.

6. The body is responding to the practitioner's statements or questions. The practitioner's *focus* directs the energy.

7. My preference for repeated muscle testing is a shoulder muscle called the pectoralis major (clavicular division), which runs from the clavicle or collarbone to the top of the humerus, the bone in the upper arm.

8. The body can only answer you by signaling "Yes" or "No," therefore you must be clear in what you are thinking, and ask it only one question per muscle test.

9. The more you practice muscle testing, the more natural it becomes.

Chapter 3

Immediate & Primal Cause

All physical ailments have varying degrees of causation, specifically, the *immediate* or most apparent cause, and the *primal*, or the root cause.

To understand the difference between immediate and primal cause, imagine you are in a vehicle, stopped at a stoplight. Suddenly, you are hit from behind by a compact car, which damages your vehicle and injures you. You manage to get out and inspect the damage. You see the compact behind you had been struck by a minivan, causing the compact to hurtle into your vehicle. Farther back, you see that a large truck struck the minivan, which struck the compact, which then hit your vehicle. The driver of the large truck is ultimately responsible for the accident.

The compact car that hit you represents the *immediate* cause. The large truck represents the *primal* cause, because that vehicle began the chain reaction.

Here's another example: Imagine someone named Michael has five brothers. Michael is going through a divorce, and he is stressed out. The oldest of his five brothers, Robert, makes fun of Michael's newly grown beard. This teasing normally would not bother Michael, but Robert is now his greatest stressor among all his brothers.

If you muscle tested Michael and asked which of his brothers was causing him the most stress, Michael's body would give you the answer that Robert is. You would have to ask the body the correct question to learn that Michael's divorce is the *primal* source of his stress, rather than his teasing brother.

More accurately, it is Michael's *emotions* about his divorce that are the primal source of his stress.

*E*motions are the primal (root) causes of our *dysfunctions, pains, intolerances, diseases and ailments.*

I am not the first to discover that emotions are the cause of all ailments, and I continue to find this through years of hands-on testing. We'll look at the power of emotions in detail in the next chapter.

The following case history illustrates perfectly the critical importance of determining the *primal* cause of dysfunctions, pains, intolerances, diseases and ailments.

Ask and You Shall Receive

When Tracy M. first came to see me, she had severe hormonal imbalance. She complained of headaches, mood changes, hot flashes, tender breasts, hair loss and frequent vaginal infections.

I identified via standard Applied Kinesiology practice the hormonal glands that were dysfunctioning, and that the thyroid gland was stressing the others. I treated her thyroid with nutrients and other Applied Kinesiology procedures.

As Tracy's thyroid gland improved, muscle testing indicated it was time to switch to treating a different hormonal gland. This helped her feel better but she was still experiencing symptoms.

One day during muscle testing, I decided to take a shortcut. Instead of asking the body which gland was the one straining the others, as is standard procedure, I asked the body what was the *cause* of the gland's dysfunction.

To my surprise, the body did not respond with another hormonal gland being the cause, as is the commonly held belief. Muscle testing indicated a dysfunction in her liver was triggering her hormonal imbalance. For months I treated her liver with nutrients and Applied Kinesiology techniques. She said she felt better than she had for years, but she still had symptoms.

Soon Tracy's condition plateaued. She grew tired of taking nutrients that upset her stomach and that she felt no longer did any good, and put her treatment on pause. A few months later, her hormonal imbalance returned, as if I'd never treated her in the first place.

I asked some of my former Applied Kinesiology teachers and mentors for advice. They all gave me variations on the well-worn phrase: "Fix what you find. That's all you can do." I appreciated their advice, but I wanted to get Tracy off this merry-go-round.

Finally it hit me. I still had not been asking a deep enough question. What I really wanted to know was what was triggering Tracy's body's imbalances in the first place. This time I asked what was the *primal* cause.

The results of my testing changed dramatically. Tracy's body indicated via muscle testing that her *emotions* were setting off a chain reaction of imbalances. Upon further questioning, I learned she had been experiencing deep grief over the death of her mother, with whom she had been extremely close.

I treated Tracy's emotions, using my Energy Healing Unlocked techniques, described in later chapters.

In Tracy's case her liver imbalance was the *immediate* cause of her hormonal imbalance. Yet it was her emotion, her grief over her mother's passing, that was the *primal* cause of all of her physical ailments.

When I asked a different question, I received a different response from the body that was much more helpful for permanent healing.

In that instant, Tracy's body illustrated to me the difference between immediate and primal causes of dysfunctions, and how important it is to understand the difference.

Immediate and Primal Causes
Chapter Summary

1. All physical ailments have varying degrees of causation, including the immediate cause and the primal cause. The primal cause is the original source.
2. Emotions are the primal causes of all our diseases, dysfunctions, pains, sensitivities and other ailments.

Chapter 4

Ruled by Our Emotions

When I first began experiencing that muscle testing always indicates emotions are the primal cause of ailments, I had a hard time
accepting this.

As a chiropractor, I have seen and experienced that adjusting
bones improves people's health and well-being. How in the world
could emotions be the cause of back pain, allergies, asthma, migraine
headaches, diabetes, tendonitis, addiction, depression, plantar fasciitis, obsessive compulsive disorder and more?

But after years of consistently and successfully correcting for
emotions as the root cause of all these ailments and more, I finally
accepted that every condition in the body has its beginnings in emotions. I can't argue with my patients' bodies — or their return to excel-
lent health.

I am not the first healer to discover how powerful emotions are.
This knowledge dates back to ancient Greece, or maybe even earlier.
Through the centuries, many physicians, psychologists, psychiatrists,
chiropractors, acupuncturists and other healers have acknowledged
that emotions exert a great influence on disease and health. Some have
even understood that emotions are the root cause of most, if not all, dis-

ease and that emotional stress worsens most diseases. However, most have not known how to use this information to help the body heal.

Emotions disrupt energy flow throughout our bodies. Energy interference causes organs, glands, muscles, ligaments and our psyche to become imbalanced and then to dysfunction, resulting in dis-ease. If emotions are traumatic enough, they can even cause genetic changes, something being studied, in part, in the field of epigenetics.

One last thought, in case you are doubting the power of our emotions. Imagine cutting a lemon in half, and squeezing the juice into your mouth. Can you feel your mouth pucker merely at the thought? Now, can you imagine the influence your thoughts have on your body when you are feeling angry, sorrowful, pressured, stressed, giddy, joyful or excited?

Sticking Her Neck Out

Cassandra came to see me with excruciating pain radiating from her neck down to the middle of her back. Conventional chiropractic care eased her pain temporarily, but it kept returning.

Cassandra explained that, for years, she had felt burdened by the self-imposed pressure to provide for all of her clients and romantic partners, regardless of how much time it took away from herself.

This pressure, a feeling of "carrying enormous weight on her shoulders," caused her to unconsciously sit at her computer in a posture jutting out her neck and chin. This placed all the weight of her head — about 10 pounds — on her cervical vertebrae, which are only designed to hold up a head when it is stacked directly above the vertebrae. This "sticking her neck out for others" turned into a chronic habit of poor posture that ultimately led to numbness down her spine and into her arms, causing sciatica from her lower back down through her legs.

Instead of adjusting the vertebrae in her neck and back, as conventional chiropractic would — and that Cassandra had tried for years, with no lasting effects — I corrected her emotional imbalance with my Energy Healing Unlocked method. Her posture became normal and her symptoms gradually disappeared.

Cassandra's story is but one of many thousands of examples I have experienced of how emotions create physical symptoms in people's bodies. When the primal cause remains untreated, symptoms can continue for a lifetime.

Primary Emotional Triggers

I have discovered there are eight primary emotional triggers that disrupt our energy flow, causing pain, dysfunction and disease. I get these primary emotional triggers 99 percent of the time while muscle testing patients' bodies. In order of frequency they are:

1. Forgiveness
2. Spiritual
3. Love
4. Over-Sympathetic
5. Mother
6. Money
7. Father
8. You

It's most efficient to muscle test in the order shown because this is the order of frequency in which these triggers appear in most people.

Ask the body in the form of a statement, either aloud or in your mind, such as, "The primary emotional trigger causing Joe's migraine headaches is 'Forgiveness.' " If the answer is "Yes," a strong muscle will weaken.

Reset the muscle to strong. Next, ask if "Forgiveness" is the *primal* emotion. If the answer is "Yes," the strong muscle will weaken, and you are ready to begin your correction. (You will learn how to make corrections in Chapter 6.)

If the answer is "No," as happens on occasion, the strong muscle will remain strong, which means you will need to delve deeper within the category of "Forgiveness" to find the *primal* emotion.

Examples of how and when this needs to be done are below, within the description of each category.

Clear Your Mind

Remember to clear your mind before you begin. Let your muscle testing allow each patient's body to tell you its story. What your logical mind believes is triggering your patient's emotions is often very different from your patient's reality.

For example, if you have a patient who was abused by her father, your logical mind might dictate that you test for anger, low self-esteem, sadness, disgust or humiliation. While muscle testing will indicate she is experiencing all of those emotions, it is probable that none of them are the primary emotional trigger.

In one patient, the primary emotional trigger might be "Forgiveness," as in "How can I ever forgive my father?" In another patient, it might be "Love," as in "How can I ever love myself enough to realize none of the abuse was my fault?"

Let muscle testing allow each patient's body to tell you its own unique truth.

Let's look at the eight primary emotional triggers in more depth.

Forgiveness

Over the course of literally hundreds of thousands of muscle tests I have done, when the body has signaled "Forgiveness" as the primary emotional trigger, I almost never have to dig deeper.

However, in case the body signals "Forgiveness" is not *primal*, here are suggestions of subcategories to muscle test:

- I need to forgive myself
- How can I forgive myself for allowing it to happen?
- I need to forgive someone else.
- I am not able to forgive.
- Someone needs my forgiveness.
- I want to be forgiven by someone.

Spiritual

The "Spiritual" category has different connotations for every person. Your patient could be seriously questioning the existence of God. They could be wrestling with guilt for not going to church when they were a child or even as an adult. They might be wrestling with which religion they should believe in, or if they should believe at all.

The beauty of this category is that you rarely need to know precisely what the issue is. The body usually responds with a "Yes" if this category is the patient's primary emotional trigger.

However, if the body gives you a "Yes" for this category, but a "No" for this category being the *primal* emotion, it is telling you to dig a bit deeper. There are myriad reasons why this could be. Use your imagination and muscle testing to test such subcategories as God, priest, rabbi, nuns, Catholic school, praying, reincarnation, etc.

Normally there is no need to ask your patient specific questions about his or her beliefs on these topics. Muscle testing the concepts themselves almost always gives you the answers you need.

For example: While muscle testing, think, " 'Reincarnation' is this patient's *primal* emotion?" If you get a "Yes," you can use "Reincarnation" to make your correction. (You will learn how to make corrections in Chapter 6.)

Love

"Love" represents all of the people and animals we have loved. If your patient's body signals that "Love" is the primary emotional trigger, but not the *primal* emotion, here is a hierarchy that is helpful to follow when delving a bit deeper:

A. Male
   a. Blood Relative
   b. In-Law
   c. Friend

B. Female
   a. Blood Relative
   b. In-Law
   c. Friend

C. Self
   a. Can't feel love
   b. Don't feel loved
   c. Don't love myself
   d. Afraid to love
   e. Too devoted
   f. Unconditional

D. Animal
   a. Cat
   b. Dog
   c. Horse
   d. Other animal

Here is how this might look when muscle testing:

1. Love (Yes, but not primal)
2. Male (No)
3. Female (No)
4. Animal (Yes, but not primal)
5. Dog (Yes, but not primal)
6. Skippy (Yes, primal)

In this example, "Love" was the primary emotional trigger, but the body indicated by muscle testing that it was not the *primal* emotion. It needed to go deeper.

Why did the body want Skippy instead of the more generic Dog? It's possible the patient had a few dogs and the body needed the exact dog with whom the patient's emotions were most deeply connected, in order to make the most complete correction. This is something you can't know in advance, but will be revealed as you muscle test.

Over-Sympathetic

"Over-Sympathetic" is a primary emotional trigger commonly found in people who are extremely sensitive. Many things bother sensitive people and they can feel hurt very easily.

For example, if a teacher tells an 8-year-old child she will never be a good student, a child who is very sensitive might develop allergies as a result of her emotional reaction to this comment. This same child could develop asthma after watching or listening to her parents argue, or seeing her mother cry afterward. Simply treating the child's asthma will help, but the asthma will have a tendency to return because the real primary emotional trigger was "Over-Sympathetic."

I've rarely had to go deeper when a patient's primary emotional trigger is "Over-Sympathetic," but here are some examples of concepts to muscle test in case the body tells you that "Over-Sympathetic" is not the *primal* emotion:

- Cry easily
- Feelings hurt
- Sensitive
- Want to go hide

Mother

I have never had the body signal that it needed anything more specific than "Mother," but if you do, you can begin muscle testing with statements such as:

- Angry at mother
- Abused by mother
- Why couldn't mother stop my abuse?
- Miss mother
- Abandoned by mother
- Want approval from mother

Money

Money is a very potent emotional trigger in our society, representing all physical things of this world. Once you get a "Yes" in this category, if the body then signals that "Money" is not the *primal* emotion, try these subcategories:

- **Cash:** Paper money and coins.
- **Bank Account:** Includes your patients' net worth, or property they own or want to own.
- **Job:** This can be a job they have, had, want or don't want. This also includes jobs that others may want them to have, or don't want them to have.
- **Career:** Can be a career they have, had, want or don't want. This includes careers others may have wanted for them, or

wish they didn't have. Example: A father wanted his son to attend college to become a doctor, but the son pursued a career as a singer. The father's deep disappointment caused emotional damage, leading to dysfunction and disease.

- **Time:** This can be a person feeling they don't have enough time to do all they want to accomplish in life, or wanting/needing more than 24 hours per day.
- **Space:** This can vary greatly. It might mean the patient feels cramped in their work or home environment. Or maybe they were forced to sleep in a closet when they were a child.

It can also be the concept of "give me my space," such as when feeling confined by another person's badgering.

Usually you will not need to delve deeply into the issues of Time or Space if the body signals that one or both are the *primal* emotion. The subcategory title is normally sufficient to correct the issues.

Here is an example of how muscle testing might look when someone's *primal* emotion is "Space."

1. Money (Yes, but not primal)
2. Space (Yes, but not primal)
3. Vehicle (Yes, primal)

This person may feel due to the price of gasoline, they have been forced to drive a compact car and they don't have enough space to feel comfortable while driving. It could extend to feeling as if they don't have enough space to even think.

It doesn't matter whether this seems logical to you. Every person is wired differently. Find the *primal* emotion, then make your correction, as instructed in Chapter 6.

Father

I have never had the body signal that it needed anything deeper than "Father," but if you do, you can begin muscle testing with statements such as:

- Angry at father
- Abused by father
- Miss their father
- Abandoned by father
- Want approval from father

You

"You" represents something a person feels about himself or herself. Although "You" seems like it would be at the top of this list, the body signals it as the primary emotional trigger less than 1 percent of the time. I don't know why this is. Perhaps the body and/or mind have incorporated typical "You" concepts into the other seven emotional triggers.

When "You" is the primary emotional trigger, it typically takes a little longer to discover than the other primary emotional triggers. Be diligent. You may need to use your intuition more in this category than in the others.

If your patient's body tells you that "You" is the primary emotional trigger, but that you need to dig deeper to find the *primal* emotion, here are some examples you can use:

- Abandoned
- Not good enough

- Afraid
- Stabbed in the back
- Alone
- Stupid
- Unappreciated, underappreciated
- Ignored
- Worthless

This is by no means a comprehensive list of what people may feel about themselves. If you are having trouble finding the *primal* emotion in this category of "You," ask the patient what they feel about themselves. You may be surprised how quickly some people will open up. Muscle test to determine which of the words is their *primal* emotion.

Case Study: Reaching

The following is an example of how "You" can work when it is the primary emotional trigger.

Ron R. had been suffering with low back pain for quite some time. He had gone to his family physician, a chiropractor and an acupuncturist and had no significant relief, so he decided to come in and check out my technique. My muscle testing confirmed his spinal pain had its roots in emotions.

I muscle tested him for the first seven primary emotional triggers, but his body indicated that none of them were at the root of his pain. Then I tested the trigger "You." The body signaled "Yes," but when I asked if "You" was *primal*, the body signaled "No."

I asked questions of his body including "You" as the son, the brother, the husband, the concept of feeling betrayed, unloved, stabbed in the back, abandoned, hurt, lonely, worthless, etc. His body signaled that none of those was his *primal* emotion for his back pain.

I put my intuition to work. I closed my eyes and felt the emotions emanating from the patient, and received the concept "Reaching." I felt as though Ron was reaching for something spiritual. He confirmed that he was searching spiritually for answers to God and for God's purpose for him."

I confirmed via muscle testing that "Reaching" was his *primal* emotion, then used "Reaching" to make the correction. Ron's low back pain disappeared after that one treatment.

Why did Ron's *primal* emotion of "Reaching" fall under "You" instead of "Spiritual?" Good question, and not one that we, as testers, can or should answer. Every person is unique.

Sugar on the Floor

Interestingly, I often receive the phrase "Sugar on the Floor" with patients for whom "You" is a *primal* emotion. Decades ago, people sprinkled sugar on the floor so that while dancing, their shoes made a crunching sound on the sugar. In energy healing, "sugar on the floor" means a person feels the best part of their lives — or the best part of them — is being stepped on, ignored, unappreciated or underappreciated.

When a patient has "You" as a primary emotion trigger, and the body signals there is more to be revealed, muscle test for the concept "sugar on the floor" and see what happens.

Free of Preconceived Notions

It is critical to keep your mind free of any preconceived notions in order to help your patients in the most effective way possible.

For example, if a client tells you they are having emotional issues stemming from a time when they were not safe in the world, or felt they were not safe, only they and their bodies know why, regardless of what you see, or what you think you know about them.

Was it because they didn't have enough money? Or because they had too much money and felt put-upon by their friends or family? Was their spouse's behavior causing them to feel that way, or was it their lack of a spouse that caused their feeling of being unsafe in the world? Was it their mother's opinions about their lack of a spouse? Could it have been their own perception of themselves? You will only know what the *primal* emotion is for each patient by muscle testing.

Feelings and Warnings

Many patients try to intellectualize or analyze their feelings while I am muscle testing. As soon as I notice this, I stop them immediately and tell them to think and feel like a 5-year-old. Have a tissue box ready because the tears usually begin to flow.

But once you have found the primary emotional trigger via muscle testing, and, if necessary, the *primal* emotion, STOP! Go no further on that topic with them. Make your correction (as described in Chapter 6), and your job is done.

It is not necessary, for example, to uncover the fact that a person's mother abandoned them when they were 5 years old. Rather, it is only necessary to discover through your muscle testing that the primary emotional trigger is "Mother."

Patients normally feel vulnerable at many stages of seeking their primary emotional trigger(s) and primal emotions. Do not encourage patients to go into more detail than you need to make corrections, unless you are a psychologist, psychiatrist or other qualified professional in a related field. If you feel it is appropriate, you can refer them to a licensed mental health professional.

Case Study: "Money"

Adele was a patient who had rheumatoid arthritis, migraine headaches and a number of other conditions. In the process of muscle testing and treating her, the primary emotional trigger of "Money" kept popping up.

The longer her body continually signaled "Money" via muscle testing, the more annoyed Adele got with me. She questioned me numerous times, verbally refuting her body's answers. I gave my usual answer: "I don't know. I just work here."

Adele told me in no uncertain terms that money could not be the issue and that I was wrong. She told me that she is wealthy, and has been wealthy all of her life. I mentioned something along the lines that maybe her mother had been poor, to which Adele immediately responded that her mother had also been wealthy all of her life. I let it go.

Suddenly, she blurted out, "I forgave her already. I'm over it already."

I couldn't help but ask, "You forgave her for what? You are over what?"

Immediately she began to cry. Adele told me that when she was 7 years old, her biological mother had traded her for a fur coat!

Now we both understood what her body had been saying all along: "Money" was indeed her primary emotional trigger.

Why had Adele's primary emotional trigger been "Money," instead of "Mother?" There is no way for us to know. Every person is emotionally wired uniquely.

Let us be grateful for this awesome tool of muscle testing God has given us, and use it to its full potential.

Note: This case took place in my earlier days when I spoke out loud to the patient what their body was answering to muscle testing. Today I simply keep the body's answers in my mind, and proceed to make the corrections.

Case Study: "Love"

Mark T. was referred to me because he was suffering from sciatica, pain that typically radiates from the lower back, down the legs, and can extend to the feet. Like many of my patients, Mark had tried physical therapy, chiropractic, prescription medication, acupuncture and more, all without any significant relief of symptoms.

Once muscle testing led us to "Emotions" as the root cause of his pain, he blurted out, "I knew it!"

He said he had been telling everyone who had been treating his sciatica, that when he was stressed, the pain intensified. He also noticed that when he was happy, or distracted by something he liked, his pain would disappear.

As I tested for his primary emotional trigger using the list of the eight triggers, his body signaled, "No" to all of them. I realized I needed to ask a different question. I asked if his primary emotional trigger was contained *within* one of the eight categories, and the body responded "Yes."

I re-tested all eight categories, with the question, "Is Mark's primary emotional trigger *within* this category?" The body signaled "No" to all except for the category of "Love."

I followed the subcategories for "Love," as shown above. Here's how it went:

1. Human (No)
2. Animal (Yes, but not primal)
3. Cat (No)
4. Dog (Yes, but not primal)
5. I asked Mark to tell me the names of all the dogs he had owned or had known. I muscle tested as he named each one. All tested as "No," until we came to Buddy.
6. Buddy (Yes, primal)

Normally at this point, you have hit pay dirt and don't need to go any further, but my intuition told me to ask just a bit more.

Mark explained that when he was a young boy, his family had to move across the country and they could not take his dog, Buddy. One day before the move, when Mark was in school, his parents gave Buddy away, and Mark never saw his dog again. With tears in his eyes, Mark told me how much he had loved Buddy and how painful it was to lose his devoted companion.

Suddenly, Mark exclaimed, "Hey, I remember I developed asthma about the same time. Do you think it had anything to do with that?" I muscle tested and his body signaled, "Yes."

After I made the correction, Mark stood up right away, saying he felt a release and a new energy in his legs. He said his pain had completely disappeared and that he could also breathe better. He kept stretching his legs, trying to make the pain return, but it would not come back. Mark said he was completely "amazed" that it could work so quickly and thoroughly.

That's the power of emotions.

Keep Your Thoughts to Yourself

Unless you are a licensed therapist, I recommend proceeding with caution when asking patients personal questions.

Additionally, as you gain proficiency, you may wish to keep most, if not all, of your questions in your mind as you are muscle testing, rather than speaking them out loud. It's equally as accurate, is certainly quicker, and minimizes the need for patients to traumatize themselves with emotional recollections. That's not required for a complete correction to be made.

However, there are times when you do need to ask more. For example, say your patient's emotional trigger is in the category "You," but the body signals that the category title of "You" is not the primal emotion. You might ask the patient an open-ended question like, "What do you think it is about the category 'You' that is your primary emotional trigger?" The patient might reply, "I feel cheated by life."

Remember, every patient is as unique as a snowflake. The vast majority of people's primary emotional triggers follow general patterns. That's why this list of eight categories is so effective. But always keep an open mind so you can help the most people possible.

As an aside, you may be wondering how I discovered these eight primary emotional triggers. It was a multi-year process via muscle testing. As you know, with muscle testing you can only receive "Yes" and "No" as answers, so I asked *lots* of questions over the years. I received the number of primary emotional triggers, what they are and the order in which they most frequently occur. Working with thousands of patients, I have found this to be true.

Ruled by Our Emotions
Chapter Summary

1. Every condition in the body has its root beginnings in emotions.
2. There are eight primary emotional triggers that interfere with our energy flow, causing pain, dysfunction and disease: Forgiveness; Spiritual; Love; Over-Sympathetic; Mother; Money; Father; You.
3. Ask the body if the emotional trigger is the *primal* emotion. If the body says "Yes" via muscle testing, this is all you need to know in order to make the correction. If the body says "No," you will need to delve deeper to find the primal emotion.

Chapter 5

Meridians & Life Energy

Now that you know how to muscle test and how to find your patient's primal emotion, your last step, before you learn how to make the correction, is to identify the manner in which this emotion is causing your patient's dysfunction. If you are not proficient in muscle testing yet, please practice more before proceeding, or you will find yourself receiving contradictory answers from the body.

According to ancient Chinese acupuncture philosophy, energy flows through channels in our body called meridians, carrying life force to every cell, organ, tissue and every system throughout our body. This energy is called by different names in different traditions, including qi or chi. I refer to it simply as energy.

The science of acupuncture — and much of Eastern medicine — associates emotions with various parts of the body, such as anger with the liver, grief with the lungs, and joy with the heart. The study of healing through acupuncture and related disciplines is much more complex than we will discuss here.

All you need to understand to use my Energy Healing Unlocked technique is that certain emotions cause energy disruption, creating imbalances in the body, thus creating various ailments or diseases. Our focus is to bring the body's energy back to its natural flow and balance.

Once you know which primal emotion is the root cause of your patient's disease, dysfunction, pain or emotional disorder, you will identify via muscle testing which meridian has had its energy disrupted by the emotion.

We will use meridian pulse points along the inside of both wrists as diagnostic points. All of the pulse points are located on the thumb side of each wrist.

Here is the list of pulse points we'll be working with (refer to image.) The words in italics are how they are referred to in various Chinese medicine modalities, followed by the body's systems/organs with which each meridian pulse point is associated:

Left wrist
1. Governing Vessel/Conception Vessel
2. *Fire*   Small Intestine/Heart
3. *Wood*   Gall Bladder/Liver
4. *Water*   Bladder/Kidney
5. Meridian
6. Meridian

Right wrist
1. Governing Vessel/Conception Vessel
2. *Metal*   Large Intestine/Lung
3. *Earth*   Stomach/Spleen
4. *Triple Heater*   Circulation/Sex Organs/Adrenals/Thyroid
5. Meridian
6. Meridian

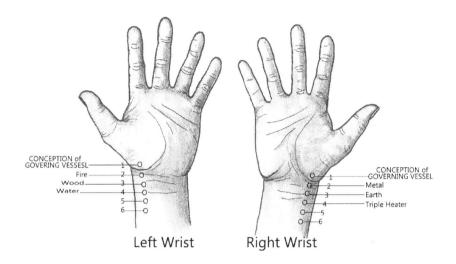

CONCEPTION of
GOVERNING VESSESL — 1
Fire — 2
Wood — 3
Water — 4
5
6

CONCEPTION of
GOVERNING VESSEL
1
Metal — 2
Earth — 3
Triple Heater — 4
5
6

Left Wrist   Right Wrist

Meridian pulse points are found along the inside (thumb side) of both wrists.

The first meridian pulse point, the Governing Vessel/Conception Vessel (GV/CV), is located at the base of the thumb, just above where the wrist bends.

Notice there are two GV/CVs, one on the meaty part of each thumb. Many healing traditions consider these to be identical, but my experience has shown me they need to be muscle tested separately. It is not important for our purposes to know how or why they are different; we simply need to be aware that they are different, then muscle test them separately from one another.

The second pulse point on each wrist begins at the bend of the wrists. The rest of the points below are separated by about the width of your fingertips, and are each about as wide as your fingertips.

You will notice that pulse points 5 and 6 are unnamed on both wrists. My experience is that these points are normally not recognized by most other healing traditions. I located them when muscle-testing the first four points on each wrist, and finding that a number of my patients' conditions were not being addressed. I have not yet named points 5 and 6, nor have I tested to find out specifically which system or organs they may be associated with, as I am not an acupuncturist, nor an expert in that science.

It is not necessary for you to memorize the names of the meridians or the organs associated with them to be able to correct dysfunctions for your patients using my Energy Healing Unlocked technique. The body will recognize the energy meridian you are testing, and will signal you, via muscles testing weak or strong, which meridian(s) you need to correct. All that is important for our purposes is to know the numbers and where these points are located.

Remember the body knows what you are thinking.

Meridians & Life Energy
Chapter Summary

1. According to ancient Chinese acupuncture philosophy, energy flows through channels in our body called meridians, carrying life force to every cell, organ, tissue and every system throughout our body.
2. There are six meridian pulse points along the inside (the thumb side) of each wrist.
3. Identify, via muscle testing, which meridian has had its energy disrupted by the emotion.

Chapter 6

Energy Healing Unlocked

Now, let's get some people well!

Begin with a picture of the meridian pulse points on the wrists in front of you (see image in prior chapter). We are going to muscle test these points in order, beginning with No. 1, continuing through to No. 6 on each wrist.

Let's say you want to correct gluten intolerance in a patient caused by the primary emotional trigger of "Money." As you know by now, when you say or think, "The primary emotional trigger of Money," and muscle test, the patient's strong muscle will become weak. Reset the muscle to strong.

Have your patient, using a finger on their right hand, touch the No. 1 pulse point on their left wrist (or you can use your own finger to touch that pulse point for them), while the patient thinks, "Money," and muscle test. If the No. 1 pulse point represents the meridian being interfered with by money, the patient's muscle will test weak. If it remains strong, continue testing pulse points 2 through 6 on the left wrist, with the patient moving their finger to each point before you test.

If none of the pulse points on the left wrist test weak (i.e. if they all test strong), continue testing on the right wrist, pulse points 1 through 6, with the patient touching those points one by one as you test, until you find the pulse point that tests weak.

You now are ready to make the correction for the patient.

Reset the muscle to strong. Have the patient touch the pulse point that caused their muscle to become weak, with a finger from their opposite hand, while you and the patient are both thinking about the emotional trigger of "Money." Simultaneously, have them place the palm of the hand with the affected pulse point, on their forehead. (This is the emotional reflex.) Have the patient continue thinking of their primary emotional trigger of "Money," holding that thought and position for two to three seconds.

Here's the critical part of this whole process: While the patient is thinking about their primary emotional trigger, *you* must also think of their pulse point and their primary emotional trigger, and "stream" that emotion to the pulse point.

Use any visual that works for you, such as seeing the emotion as steam, pouring it on as if it was liquid or physically pasting that emotional trigger onto the pulse point. Send that emotional trigger to the pulse point in whatever way feels most effective for you.

Reset the muscle to strong, then muscle test for the condition that you were attempting to correct, such as gluten intolerance. If the muscle remains strong, you have corrected the patient's gluten intolerance.

If the muscle weakens again, reset the muscle to strong, then re-test the primary emotional triggers (Chapter 4) and pulse points (Chapter 5).

Sometimes, in order to correct a condition, multiple emotional triggers and pulse points need to be addressed. Keep re-testing and making corrections until the body signals, via muscle testing, that the condition has been cleared.

Here is a sample muscle testing script for making corrections, using the example of correcting gluten intolerance.

1. Say or think, "Gluten intolerance," while muscle testing. If the person is gluten intolerant, the strong muscle will weaken. Reset the muscle to strong.
2. Muscle test through the eight primary emotional triggers.
3. Say or think, "Forgiveness." Muscle stays strong.
4. Say or think, "Spiritual." Muscle stays strong.
5. Say or think, "Love." Muscle stays strong.
6. Say or think, "Over-Sympathetic." Muscle weakens. "Over-Sympathetic" is your primary emotional trigger. Reset the muscle to strong.
7. Say or think, "Over-Sympathetic" while either you or the patient touches their left No. 1 pulse point. Muscle stays strong.
8. Say or think, "Over-Sympathetic, left wrist, No. 2 pulse point," while either you or the patient touches their left No. 2 pulse point. Muscle stays strong.
9. Say or think, "Over-Sympathetic, left wrist, No. 3 pulse point," while either you or the patient touches their left No. 3 pulse point. Muscle stays strong. Continue testing pulse points 4, 5 and 6 on the left. Let's assume for this example that when testing pulse points 4, 5 and 6, the muscle stays strong.
10. Say or think, "Over-Sympathetic, right wrist, No. 1 pulse point" while either you or the patient touches their right No. 1 pulse point. Let's assume the muscle weakens. This is the pulse point that has an imbalance you are going to correct.

11. Reset the muscle to strong.

12. Have the patient touch their GV/CV point with their left index finger, and bring the palm of their right hand to their forehead, while thinking "Over-Sympathetic." Both of you hold this thought for several seconds, sending thoughts of "Over-Sympathetic" to the right No. 1 GV/CV point.

13. Muscle test again for gluten intolerance. Muscle stays strong. Gluten intolerance corrected!

Just a reminder that having the patient touch places on their body is merely your visual aid to help you keep your focus on each and every specific question you are asking the body. If your mind wanders, or if you rely on the patient's hand placements more than on your focus, the answers you receive via muscle testing will be inaccurate. Remember to stream the emotion to the meridian or to the heart so the correction will take place.

A word of caution about correcting food intolerances: I always advise patients to take things slowly after treatment, especially if someone has had severe allergies, such as if their breathing has become restricted or they have had to be hospitalized after eating certain substances. I actually advise people who have had more severe reactions never to eat that food again — or to do so only with extreme caution, and to make sure they have their EpiPen (a medical device for injecting a measured dose or doses of epinephrine, a chemical that narrows blood vessels and opens airways in the lungs), or similar remedy nearby.

Remember, as with most, if not all, types of healing procedures, you have provided the patient with healing energy, but what they do after they leave your office is beyond your control. Emotional triggers can return under stress, recreating intolerances or dysfunctions.

Fine Tuning: Multiple Pulse Points

On rare occasions, you may find that none of the 12 pulse points will muscle test weak. This means that more than one pulse point is affected by the primary emotional trigger. The body won't specify only one, because to obtain correction, you will need to work with two pulse points at the same time.

There are two ways to determine which two meridians are affected:

1. Muscle test one pulse point at a time, asking the body, "Is this one of the two?" - or -

2. Touch two pulse points at once while muscle testing and asking the body, "Are these the two points?" You will need to try various combinations.

For example, you might have to have the patient think "Money," while having them touch both the Wood and Water pulse points at once (point numbers 3 and 4 on the left wrist).

Also, I have never found two pulse points needing correction that were separated by another pulse point in between; the two have always been side-by-side. Nor have I found a pulse point on one wrist and another pulse point on the other wrist needing correction to clear a condition. But you might experience such a circumstance, as all patients are unique.

Corrections: Questions & Answers

Here are some common questions when people are learning my Energy Healing Unlocked technique.

Q: What should I feel when making the correction?

A: Most people feel a shift in energy. This becomes more noticeable over time, as you become more sensitive to energy. You may feel a sense of completion, a sense of knowing, similar to the way in which you know your own name. At times, you may feel the energy in the patient's muscle weakening even before you actually put any pressure on their muscle. In time, you will develop this degree of sensitivity and intuition.

Q: How can I tell if I actually made the correction?

A: Muscle test for the condition you are trying to correct. If the muscle remains strong, you have completed this correction.

If the muscle weakens, reset the muscle to strong, and repeat the correction. Re-test for the condition again.

If the muscle weakens again, do not assume that you did something wrong. Often it means an imbalance needs more correction on deeper levels, such as discovering additional primary emotional triggers.

Q: I think I found the proper pulse point to correct, but how can I be sure?

A: Ask the body via muscle testing. Often when people are learning my Energy Healing Unlocked technique, they will confirm the pulse points two or three times before beginning their correction.

Q: I thought I knew what my patient's primary emotional triggers were going to be, but none of them muscle tested as "Yes."

A: Keep your mind clear before, during and after your testing, and, of course, while making corrections. You need to be a clear conduit so the body can tell you what it needs you to know, rather than what you *think* you know.

Further, hold only one thought in your mind at a time, as the body can only answer one question at a time. If you are holding multiple thoughts i.e. asking multiple questions of the body at once, you will receive inaccurate answers.

Q: I am having trouble finding which pulse point(s) to perform the correction on.

A: You may have inadvertently broken the chain of thinking somewhere along the line. Re-test from the beginning.

Q: A small group of us have been practicing on a friend, who is serving as our "patient." Several of us are getting different primary emotional triggers. Is anyone doing anything wrong? Is our patient tricking us?

A: The beauty of muscle testing is that the body can't lie, regardless of what your patient wants the answers to be! Different emotions and/or pulse points can be indicated at different times by the body. Emotions have many layers and dimensions, each being revealed when the patient's body is ready to release them.

Q: Is it possible for me as the practitioner to do all the streaming of thoughts to the pulse points? If so, is it really necessary for me or the patient to touch their pulse points while I am doing the correction?

A: Great question! Yes, you as the practitioner are able to do all the streaming of thoughts to the pulse points *without* the patient's help, and without either of you touching the pulse points. This is your ultimate goal. It is just as accurate and many times faster.

However, I recommend that you continue touching or having the patient touch the pulse points until you become adept at making corrections. You will know when you are able to hold your focus clearly and strongly enough that you are able to discontinue actually touching the pulse points, and instead merely think of them. Muscle testing will confirm if you have made the corrections.

Shortcut: Straight to the Heart

I recently discovered a shortcut for making corrections. Instead of muscle testing each meridian pulse point, one day I asked the body, "Is there a master controller?" Through muscle testing, the body indicated the heart is the meridian controller.

Here's how this shortcut works. Muscle test to find the primary emotional trigger. Reset the muscle to strong. Then, ask the body if the imbalance can be corrected via the patient's heart, instead of the pulse points.

If the body indicates "Yes," via a weak muscle, reset the muscle to strong, stream that emotion to the person's heart, then muscle test again to confirm the correction has been made.

This shortcut can certainly save you time, though it's necessary that you become proficient making corrections with the pulse points, for there are times when the body doesn't allow you to go straight to the heart. Every patient is unique.

One Step at a Time

Although these techniques sound simple, it can take a lot of practice before becoming proficient in them. Do not give up! Simply take things one step at a time. It will be worth all the time you invest. Once you perform corrections a few times and find out how much better your patients are feeling, I guarantee you will be overwhelmingly filled with joy.

If you are feeling challenged in grasping how to heal with energy, remember that all of the concepts I am presenting in this book are different ways of thinking from any you may have encountered in your life, until now. Becoming proficient in energy healing has nothing to do with intelligence. It's purely adjusting to a new mindset — and practice, practice, practice.

Remember, ANYONE can do energy healing, not just a chosen few. It may come more naturally to some people than to others, but that's why practice is important. We are all healers.

Powerful Medicine

If you follow these procedures correctly, the vast majority of your patients will feel better after their first treatment. Most of your patients will remain corrected for years and not have to return for periodic treatments, unless they re-subject themselves to the emotional conditions that caused their imbalances originally.

However, since every disease has its roots in emotions, and we are, if nothing else, emotional beings, your patients can reactivate their dysfunctions by following old patterns of behavior and thought. Some people will need to be treated periodically to manage their conditions for awhile. In most cases, every time you correct a condition, the intensity and the severity will decrease. (More in Chapter 15 about simple, yet vital, techniques to help your patients keep their emotionally-based dysfunctions from recurring.)

This is designed to minimize ongoing treatment, because you have accessed the root cause.

Energy Healing Unlocked

As you become adept at using my Energy Healing Unlocked technique, you will find this procedure corrects conditions and diseases faster than any other healing method you have ever heard of or tried. Once you become proficient, it usually takes only several seconds to make each correction.

Through my Energy Healing Unlocked system we are simply removing the emotional stumbling blocks that were once interfering with patients' bodies' natural healing mechanisms.

Energy Healing Unlocked
Chapter Summary

1. Muscle test the meridian pulse points in order, beginning with No. 1, continuing through to No. 6 on each wrist.

2. When you find the meridian pulse point on which the strong muscle tests weak, reset the muscle to strong.

3. Have the patient touch that pulse point with a finger from their opposite hand. Simultaneously, have them place the palm of the hand with the affected pulse point, on their forehead, holding that thought and position for several seconds, while they think about their primary emotional trigger, and while you "Stream" that emotion to the pulse point.

4. Muscle test again for the condition you are trying to correct. If the muscle tests strong, you have corrected that condition.

5. If the muscle tests weak, reset the muscle to strong, and re-correct.

6. If the muscle still tests weak, reset it to strong and retest all eight primary emotional triggers, then pulse points. Sometimes emotional triggers and pulse points need to be corrected more than once.

7. Once the body signals via a strong muscle, the cause of the condition has been corrected.

8. Once you become proficient, you as the practitioner are able to do all the streaming of thoughts to the pulse points without the patient's help, and without either of you touching the pulse points. It is just as accurate and many times faster.

9. A shortcut is going straight to the heart instead of the pulse points, because the heart is the meridian controller. Muscle test to determine if this can be done. Sometimes the body won't allow the correction to be made through the heart. Every patient is unique.

Chapter 7

Faster Than a Speeding Bullet

As you progress, your patients' bodies will automatically know when you are ready to graduate to the next level, as happened when Betty S. flew in from another state for treatment for gluten intolerance.

After spending quite a bit of time listening to Betty speak, I saw I was running out of time before my next patient was going to arrive. I quickly muscle tested Betty, without explaining to her what I was doing. I found her primary emotional trigger and which pulse point was responsible. Unbeknownst to me, the moment I learned which pulse point needed to be rebalanced, the body corrected itself!

Right before repeating the testing more slowly, so I could explain to Betty what I was doing, and *before* I instructed her to touch her pulse points and her emotional reflex on her forehead, I decided to demonstrate to her again, via muscle testing, that she was gluten intolerant. I placed a small container of flour on her abdomen, just as I had done earlier in our session. Normally her strong muscle would weaken — but this time it stayed strong. I figured I must not have been concentrating well on the flour, so I tested again, and several more times. But her muscle that would have weakened with the gluten was now staying strong.

I did not know what to think. I don't even remember what I told her, probably something like, "In the process of testing I must have corrected the gluten intolerance ahead of time," not realizing how close to the truth this was.

I was perplexed. Why did her gluten intolerance correct before I had her go through the correction procedure with me?

As I continued treating other patients for various dysfunctions, the same thing happened from time to time: Conditions were correcting themselves before I manually went through the correction procedure with each patient. I knew corrections had definitely been made, because all of the patients were able to eat the foods they had previously been intolerant to, or their dysfunctions cleared up.

After it happened for the sixth or seventh time, I realized that as I muscle tested, the healing was taking place, before I had a chance to go through the correction procedures. Merely by my thinking or envisioning the dysfunction, the emotion and the meridian pulse points and/or heart, the body was making the corrections.

*Y*our focus directs the healing energy.

One day I asked the body, "Who is doing the healing, the doctor or the patient? The body signaled, "The doctor."

I was almost scared at what I had just heard.

Then I realized it is via our focus that God, the Universe or whatever higher power you ascribe to, directs the healing energy.

I proceeded muscle testing patients, and instead of having my patients touch their wrist pulse points and their foreheads, I simply *thought* of the pulse points and the primary emotional triggers by myself. I no longer needed the patients' help. Each patient's body functioned as my visual aid, keeping my focus.

All the conditions and diseases I was correcting for patients, such as allergies, rheumatoid arthritis, muscle weakness and lower back pain, were disappearing simply with my thinking of the primary emotional triggers and the pulse points. Many of my patients would say while on my treatment table, "I can feel the pain and swelling going down," or "I can feel the energy flowing."

Conditions and diseases were getting better, faster than a speeding bullet, and the results were longer lasting. Most of my patients' conditions never returned and no further treatments were required.

Jumping the Gap

I was being led, via muscle testing, directly from the condition or ailment, to the primary emotional trigger that was causing the condition, literally "jumping the gap" from the dysfunction to the emotion, without having to identify any conditions in between.

My patients were getting well even faster than before. To me, the name of the game is to help patients heal with as few treatments as possible.

Of course, I wished I had thought of this sooner! But the body wouldn't have led me there any sooner than I was ready to understand this was possible.

The entire learning process is similar to teaching a child the mechanics of swimming while they are standing on dry land, beside a swimming pool. After doing so, if I were to toss that child into the water and tell her to swim, she more than likely would not be able to do it. She wouldn't have the ability, nor confidence that it is possible.

That's why we give kids life jackets, so they can remain safely afloat while learning.

In time, as you gain experience, you will be able to "jump the gap" yourself, and rely solely on energy healing.

Patience, Grasshopper

You might be thinking, "Why didn't he tell us how to jump the gap in the first place?"

Without understanding the principles of why muscles weaken or stay strong during muscle testing, how to think, what to think, the difference between an immediate cause and primary cause, primary emotional triggers, primal emotions, energy meridians and pulse points, you would have been unable to hold the line of thought the body requires to make corrections.

You also might have thought this is too fantastic to be believed, unless you had come along on this journey with me, as you now have done.

If you are wondering how I figured all this out, rest assured, I did not do it on my own. I have always asked God for answers, and have always been provided them for the help I can give others.

Faster Than a Speeding Bullet
Chapter Summary

1. Once your mental focus becomes laser sharp, your testing time may dramatically decrease, as the energy begins to flow more rapidly from your mind to the patient's body.
2. Your focus directs the healing energy.

Chapter 8

Diseases,
Putting the Body on Autopilot
& Sequential Healing

If you have understood the concepts I have described up to this point, and if you have been practicing your muscle testing technique, you have all of the tools necessary to correct any condition or dysfunction a person may have that is causing a disease.

However, with diseases, there are often multiple layers.

Have you ever heard of someone who was told by a physician that they had a particular disorder, then was told by another doctor they were suffering from something else, then a third physician came up with a third diagnosis? Guess what? All three doctors were probably correct! The person was likely suffering from multiple conditions. But in many disciplines, we are trained to ask, "What does this patient have?" We should be asking, "What things does this patient have?"

For example, if a patient comes to see me because they have rheumatoid arthritis (an autoimmune disease), but is unaware she also suffers from lupus (another autoimmune disease), I could correct the cause of the rheumatoid arthritis, but the patient's symptoms caused by lupus would remain. In my experience, most patients who have an autoimmune disease are also suffering from some degree of another autoimmune disease, such as lupus, fibromyalgia or Hashimoto's disease.

So, how can we correct something we don't yet know exists in our patients' bodies? Begin by testing for conditions you know the patient has, or they have told you they have.

Then continue searching for conditions that neither you, nor the patient, are aware they have, using a list of diseases segregated by category. It's easiest to begin with the World Health Organization's disease classification system, which is summarized in 10 broad areas. There is a degree of overlap in this list. For example, cancer can fall into more than one of these categories, but this list is a great help.

- Heart, Lung and Other Organ Diseases
- Blood and Immune System Diseases
- Cancer
- Injury
- Brain and Nervous System Diseases
- Endocrine System Diseases
- Infectious and Parasitic Diseases
- Pregnancy and Childbirth-Related Diseases
- Inherited Diseases
- Environmentally-Acquired Diseases

Unless a disease is solely hereditary or caused by an environmental issue, there normally is more than one emotional trigger that caused the imbalance or dysfunction. I have found that when correcting for diseases, you may return to the same one or two emotional trigger categories multiple times.

Simply go down the list, muscle testing by category until you find the primary emotional trigger, and the corresponding pulse point(s) that need to be corrected, as described in previous chapters.

However, there is an easier, quicker way, described in the next section.

Sequential Healing:
Putting the Body on Autopilot

One day, I was treating a patient named David for knee pain. With only two minutes left before my next patient arrived, David asked if I would treat his shoulder. Wanting to help, but feeling in a rush, I asked his body to fix the most important thing in the patient's shoulder. Then I asked it to fix the second-most important thing in his shoulder. I quickly muscle tested to find the primary emotional trigger associated with each of those things, muscle tested for the pulse points, and did the correction.

Almost immediately, David said his shoulder was feeling better. When he returned a week later, he said his shoulder was much improved.

Once I realized what had happened with David, I began asking other patients' bodies to correct the *most important* things first, then the second, then the third most important, etc., regardless whether or not I knew what those things were. To my surprise, each of their bodies responded, via muscle testing, that every ailment I could think of, was being corrected.

I had inadvertently learned that we can put a body on autopilot and allow it to heal itself in the order it deems best.

By putting the body on autopilot, we instruct the body to correct the most important thing first, and to continue correcting sequentially.

When we place the body on autopilot and tell it to heal itself sequentially, it is smart enough to heal things in the order that makes the most sense for itself. It will automatically advance from the first most important thing, to the second most important thing, then the third most important thing, etc. The body will signal, via your muscle testing, when it is done.

By allowing the body to go on autopilot, we can also prevent worse things from happening.

For example, say you have a patient who complains of pain in her right knee. Unbeknownst to her she is also suffering from cardiovascular disease and inflammation. By placing the body on autopilot and sequential healing, the body can correct the cardiovascular issues before the knee pain, saving the patient from a probable heart attack.

Most importantly, when we let a body heal itself on autopilot, via sequential healing, it addresses issues that might have taken us a long time to discover.

When I first began muscle testing, I used to have a list of every muscle, ligament, tendon, bursa, cartilage, disease and condition I could think of, and I would test for them all. By doing so, I unknowingly controlled the body by restricting it to the options on my list, and to the order in which I was testing. I hadn't realized I was limiting what the body could do.

Now that we know we can heal via autopilot, the body is free to heal all that it knows needs to be healed, in the order it knows is most effective.

Visualize

When doing sequential healing, your ability to visualize can come in handy. I either envision the patient's body as a totem pole, or as a roll of salami standing on one end, in preparation for slicing in a delicatessen meat-slicing machine.

When I test for the first condition (I don't know what the condition is; I am letting the body figure that out), I start at the top of the totem pole and visualize myself climbing down with each correction. Alternately, I visualize the body as a salami I am slicing, from top to bottom.

Here's how the muscle testing might look when using sequential healing and placing the body on autopilot. Let's assume the patient tells you she has fibromyalgia and Hashimoto's disease, but she may also have additional autoimmune diseases that haven't been medically diagnosed.

1. Begin with a strong muscle.
2. Think "Autoimmune disease."
3. Muscle will weaken if patient has *any* autoimmune disease. Reset the muscle to strong.
4. Think the concept, "I want every autoimmune disease in this body fixed."
5. Now test for the primary emotional trigger. Let's say "Forgiveness" is the primary emotional trigger that causes the muscle to weaken. Reset the muscle to strong.
6. Now test the wrist pulse points, one by one, or the heart if the body will allow it, as described in Chapter 6.
7. When you find the pulse point on which the muscle weakens, reset the muscle to strong, then "stream" or energetically send that emotion to that point.
8. Muscle test again for autoimmune diseases. We do this again because normally if a patient has an autoimmune disease, they have more than one and/or other dysfunctions.

9. If the muscle tests weak for autoimmune diseases again, reset the muscle to strong, then repeat the process of testing for the patient's primary emotional trigger. The body is on autopilot, and will let you know via muscle testing when there are more autoimmune diseases and/or dysfunctions to test for, and correct.

10. When the muscle tests strong for autoimmune diseases, you are complete.

It may take multiple rounds of finding and correcting primary emotional triggers to correct for autoimmune diseases. Normally a patient has experienced more than one emotional issue that contributed to their autoimmune condition.

You can perform the same sequential healing/autopilot procedure for any ailment, not only for diseases. For example, when a patient has a rotator cuff problem, I tell the body to correct the most important thing in the shoulder first, then second, etc. until the body signals via muscle testing that there is nothing else wrong in the patient's shoulder area.

This works because over the years, I have instructed the body to fix "everything wrong with this shoulder area," which encompasses every muscle, ligament, structure, tendon, inflammation, disease, autoimmune condition, arthritis, pain or any other ailment that is involved in that shoulder.

As I have said before: the power lies in *how* you are thinking and *what* you are thinking. It's your laser-like focus that directs the healing energy.

"I feel like a new person!"

When I was first learning how to place patients' bodies on auto-pilot, Stephen R. came to see me, explaining that he had symptoms that included numbness, body stiffness, muscle and body shaking, and muscle spasms. Via muscle testing, I instructed his body to start correcting imbalances or dysfunctions beginning with the most important, then to continue making corrections to increasingly minor issues.

Within about 20 minutes, Stephen's body signaled via muscle testing that it was done. To make sure, I muscle tested every structure, organ and reflex condition on his body that I could think of. His body indicated that *everything* had been corrected. I told Stephen to return in one week.

During that week, I continued treating patients by putting their bodies on autopilot, asking their bodies to sequentially correct all that was needed.

One week later, Stephen returned to my office and told me, "I feel like a new person." Other patients' comments were almost identical: "I don't know what you did to me but I feel great!" My patients with neurological issues and other conditions reported that their symptoms had disappeared.

"Anything Wrong"

Putting the body on autopilot to heal itself sequentially was working so well for my patients, that one day, I decided to take things even further. I asked a patient's body, via muscle testing, if the person had "anything wrong" with them, structurally, a disease, a dysfunction, an emotional or mental condition. Unless you are testing Superman, any body will respond with a "Yes," via muscle testing, because practically everybody has something that is dysfunctioning in them, even if very minor.

Here is how muscle testing "anything wrong" can look:

1. Begin with a strong muscle.
2. Think, "Anything wrong with this body?" and muscle test. If the muscle tests weak, reset the muscle to strong.
3. Think, "Begin with the most important first." Muscle test.
4. The muscle will weaken, signaling the body acknowledges the first dysfunction to correct.
5. Reset the muscle to strong. Then muscle test for the primary emotional trigger(s) causing the first dysfunction, resetting the muscle to strong after each answer that weakens it.
6. Muscle test for the pulse point(s), or the heart if the body will allow it, that will correct the primary emotional trigger(s), resetting the muscle to strong after each answer that weakens it.
7. Perform the corrections as described in Chapter 6.

Next, repeat the steps above while directing the body to look for the second, third and fourth most important conditions or dysfunctions. Remember, when healing sequentially, the body knows what to fix, in the most beneficial order.

Use your visualization of the body as a totem pole, a roll of salami, or whatever imagery works for you.

You will know when the body has completed all of its corrections when you muscle test a strong muscle with the statement: "Anything wrong with this body," and the muscle remains strong.

I perform sequential and autopilot healing on every patient on every visit. Done correctly, it only takes several minutes.

Healing sequentially is similar to aiming a bowling ball down the alley: When you strike the first pin accurately, all the remaining pins fall without any additional effort on your part.

Write It Down

If visualizing is challenging for you, you can write on a sheet of paper: "Anything wrong with the body," and muscle test for the concept while looking at the paper, following the same steps as above. This will work no matter what language you write it in, as long as you as the tester, know what is written on that piece of paper, and focus on it.

Let the body and the Universe read your mind.

Symptoms

When a person has been diagnosed with a disease, they normally have been experiencing an assortment of very unpleasant symptoms. After you have made your corrections on the patient's body via my Energy Healing Unlocked system, some patients will notice a difference immediately. For others, it may take some time.

As patients begin to feel better, some may ask you if they should continue taking their doctor-prescribed medication. Advise your patients to speak to their doctor.

Never interfere with your patients' relationship with their physician, nor with anything their physician may have prescribed for them.

Energy healing works in conjunction with Western medicine, healing energetic blocks to physical healing.

Diseases,
Putting the Body on Autopilot
& Sequential Healing
Chapter Summary

1. Testing and correcting for diseases is performed the same way we test and correct for all other conditions.

2. When correcting the root cause of diseases, be aware that patients can have multiple conditions.

3. Muscle test until you find the primary emotional trigger, and the corresponding pulse point(s) that need to be corrected, or the heart, if the body will allow it, as described in previous chapters.

4. We can put a body on autopilot and allow it to heal itself sequentially, instructing the body to correct the most important thing first, then the second most important thing, then the third most important thing, etc., and to keep going until the body signals, via muscle testing, that all have been corrected.

Chapter 9
Mental Disorders & Addiction

Testing for and correcting the imbalances that have caused mental disorders and conditions is performed the same way we test and correct for all other conditions. If you have understood the concepts I have described up to this point, and if you have been practicing your muscle testing technique, you have all the tools necessary to correct any condition or dysfunction a person may have that is causing a mental disorder.

I have experienced that when patients come to me with conditions such as depression, addiction, bipolar disorder, dyslexia, obsessive-compulsive disorder, among others, that they usually have additional mental and/or emotional conditions they might not know they have. Unless you correct all of them, the patient can continue to suffer mentally and emotionally.

Accordingly, it is best to muscle test your patient for multiple mental disorders. It's easiest to begin by creating a list from a basic search online of all known mental disorders. Also include emotional issues such as phobias, self-hatred and self-destruction. Simply go down the list, muscle test and correct for each one of them.

Better yet, when you feel ready to work faster and more comprehensively, instruct the body to correct sequentially "all mental and emotional conditions."

When I do this, at least 50 percent of my patients tell me while still on my treatment table that they feel a difference while I am making my way down the list and making corrections!

Correcting imbalances that cause mental disorders is best illustrated through the following examples.

Depression

Robert C. was referred to me because he was suffering from severe clinical depression. When I have a patient who is aware they are suffering from depression, I always have them rate their depression on a scale from 0 to 10, with 0 being happy, with no conscious knowledge of them being depressed, and 10 being seriously contemplating suicide or having attempted suicide in the past.

Robert stated he was a 10. Not only had he previously attempted suicide, but it was still lingering in his mind. He said he was under the care of a psychologist and a psychiatrist, the latter of whom had prescribed antidepressant medication. He said he felt he was wasting his time with both professionals, because his psychologist told him they were going to be "friends for a long time" and his psychiatrist kept giving him different pills that made him feel worse and "less connected to the world." He was discouraged that no one seemed interested in helping him get well. He felt there was no end in sight.

I began my treatment by first identifying and getting an acknowledgement from the body that he had depression, because quite often this is medically misdiagnosed.

Through muscle testing, his body signaled that Robert was indeed suffering from depression. The second step was to identify the primary emotional trigger responsible for his depression. The third step was to identify the meridian that was being affected by the primary emotional trigger. Once I identified all three factors, I made the correction. Robert, having never been to see me before, didn't know what I was doing.

Within two to three seconds of making the correction, he said, "Wow, what a rush!"

He said he could actually feel the energy flowing through his body, and that he felt a wave of happiness wash through his body.

After I finished my treatment, I asked him to return in several days. You never know what can happen between visits with patients who have severe depression, so I wanted only a short time between his first few treatments.

A few days later, Robert returned to my office. He rated his depression on the 0 to 10 scale at 0! I was so taken aback by his dramatic improvement, I had to ask him to repeat himself. Again, he said "0!"

He said he no longer had thoughts of suicide.

Then he began to cry. He said that for the first time in many years, he felt absolutely no depression.

"I finally understand the saying, 'High on life.' Before this, I never quite understood how or why people could be so happy," he said. "I must have had depression all my life, because I have never felt as good as I do right now."

Addiction

Serafin was 22 years old and suffering from addiction to alcohol and street drugs. He said he had been to two drug rehabilitation centers and Alcoholics Anonymous, but the programs helped him only temporarily because he still had the desire to drink and take drugs. His mother had heard about me, so they decided to give me a try.

The first question Serafin's mother asked me was, "How could a chiropractor help my son get off drugs and quit drinking?" I explained to them that addiction is like being on a merry-go-round, wanting to get off but not being able to. I also explained that emotional stress on Serafin's body was disrupting his energy, creating his addictive personality.

I explained how muscle testing works, then quickly demonstrated how weak muscles on Serafin strengthened within seconds after energy healing. They were both excited to get started.

I began by confirming via muscle testing that Serafin indeed had an addictive personality. I identified the primary emotional trigger responsible, then identified the meridian whose energy was being blocked by that trigger. Then I made the correction by visualizing the meridian pulse points affected and mentally "streaming" the primary emotional trigger to the meridian pulse point, just as I have described earlier in this book.

Within seconds, Serafin began to cry. He said he felt a release in his body and mind, as though he had finally been released from a horrible emotional prison.

When Serafin and his mother returned a week later, he said he no longer felt the need to drink alcohol or take drugs. Because he had been able to stop, Serafin felt free.

When treating patients with substance abuse or other addictive issues, be sure to test for, and correct, all aspects of their addiction. There are three major aspects, though with some patients, you may find more.

- **Addictive Personality**: Wanting to stop or get off the merry-go-round, but being unable to;
- **Physical Addiction**: Their body "knowing" it needs this substance;
- **Emotional Addiction**: Fear of stopping, such as feeling if they discontinue drinking or doing drugs, they will need to face traumatic memories, social anxiety or societal pressures.

All three aspects must be corrected for the patient to be able to return fully to his or her normal balance.

Here is the abridged version of my script for treating Serafin:

1. I started with a strong muscle.
2. I thought "Addictive Personality," and muscle tested. Serafin's muscle tested weak. I reset the muscle to strong.
3. I muscle tested for the primary emotional trigger of "Love." The muscle tested weak. I reset the muscle to strong.
4. When I muscle tested the pulse points on his wrists, the Number 1 pulse point on his left wrist, the GV/CV, tested weak.
5. I reset the muscle to strong, then streamed emotion of "Love" to his left wrist, the Number 1 pulse point.
6. I re-muscle tested "Addictive Personality," and the muscle remained strong. That was his body's way of saying the "Addictive Personality" was corrected.
7. I repeated the process for "Physical Addiction" and "Emotional Addiction."

Multiple Personalities

Glenn came to see me for an array of issues, including multiple personality disorder. He asked me to correct his physical conditions first. On his third visit, which we had agreed would be his last, I was ready to relieve him of his multiple personalities. However, he said, "I've changed my mind. I've decided that I don't want you to fix that now."

Puzzled, I asked why he did not want me to correct the disorder. "I like her," he said, "and I don't think I want to give her up yet."

Confused, I asked, "Who is it you don't want to give up?"

He said, "You know — *her.*"

I was baffled. Did he have a girlfriend I had forgotten about? So, I asked again, "I'm sorry. Who are you talking about?"

"You know, my other friend," he said.

I now realized he was talking about his other personality, whom I had never spoken to, and this personality was female. Apparently, he found comfort in her, and he wanted to keep her around for a while.

His attitude surprised me, but it was his right to decline treatment. I would correct the multiple personality disorder if and when he was ready.

A few months later he returned to my office to correct the disorder. He was ready to let go of his female friend. I made the correction, and Glenn has not had any other personality return.

Glenn later told me that he did not think I'd be able to correct any of his physical or mental ailments at all. His parents had insisted he see me because they had heard about my treatment method. When he realized my technique was actually ridding him of his physical conditions, he had feared that he might not have been able to function without his "friend."

He said he found great comfort in the fact I did not pressure him to get rid of his friend before he was ready to let her go. He thanked me for respecting his wishes and giving him power to control his own healing.

Mental Disorders
Chapter Summary

1. Testing for and correcting the imbalances that have caused mental disorders and conditions is performed the same way we test and correct for all other conditions.

2. Create a list from a basic search online of all known mental disorders, including emotional issues such as phobias, self-hatred, self-destruction, etc., then muscle test.

3. To correct for addiction, you need to muscle test for, and correct the patient's addictive personality, physical addiction and emotional addiction.

Chapter 10

Emotional Intolerances

Some time ago I was reading a book in which a psychiatrist using kinesiological muscle testing claimed you could muscle test to determine whether a patient was compatible with his or her mate, or the person they were considering dating.

This intrigued me, because many times my patients complain about their significant other, how unhappy they are with this person, and how this creates stress in their life. I decided to find out how my Energy Healing Unlocked system might apply in such a condition.

When two people who were once compatible now find themselves incompatible, one or both of them may have developed emotional or mental issues, such as narcissism, bipolar/manic-depressive disorder, depression or attention deficit/hyperactivity disorder.

We have the tools to correct these issues, and it can literally be life-changing for your patient.

The beauty of this procedure is you do not have to identify who or what the problem is. Simply envision the two people together, and intend that if they are emotionally intolerant to each other, the strong muscle will weaken when you muscle test.

Treat emotional intolerances as though you were attempting to correct a food intolerance. Simply test the eight primary emotional triggers, resetting the muscle to strong each time an answer weakens it, and making the corrections as described in Chapter 6.

After making the first correction (and resetting the muscle to strong), re-envision the two people together. If a strong muscle continues to weaken, there are other issues to correct. Continue testing and correcting until the body signals all is corrected, via the muscle remaining strong when you envision the two people together.

Typically, my patients return in about a week thanking me, telling me their significant other seems to be a different person and that they are getting along much better now.

This technique can also be used for parent-child emotional intolerances, and for emotional intolerances among friends.

Here are steps for addressing an emotional tolerance issue between two people:

1. Visualize a person in a container on your patient's abdomen.
2. Muscle test. If the strong muscle weakens, his/her body is stating the two people are not compatible.
3. Reset the muscle to strong. Think of the two people together, then muscle test to find the primary emotional trigger responsible for the intolerance, remembering to reset the muscle to strong each time an answer weakens it. When the strong muscle weakens, you have found the primary emotional trigger(s).
4. Muscle test for the meridian pulse point(s) involved, or the heart if the body will allow it, and make your correction as described in Chapter 6.

Mother and Baby

I have discovered via muscle testing that a pregnant mother can be either physically or emotionally intolerant to the fetus, or both. The body has also indicated via muscle testing that a fetus, while in the womb, can be intolerant to itself.

Interestingly, I have discovered that you can correct intolerance(s) in both the mother and the fetus, but there are times when you may need to also address imbalances or a dysfunction in the placenta, otherwise it can act as a barrier between the mother and fetus.

You don't need to know why these intolerances, imbalances or dysfunctions exist. You can simply correct them for your patient using the technique above.

Disclaimer

Please understand that one or two treatments does not necessarily correct all of the issues that two people may have with each other. Their patterns of behavior may take awhile to change, so you may need to perform multiple corrections. Every relationship is unique.

This technique works only when you expect it to work, and likewise expect the body to respond accordingly. If you have doubts, you will be sending energetic frequencies that are the opposite of corrections, and your work will not be as effective.

Further, this technique only corrects the issues that make these two people incompatible with each other. In order to correct other personal issues that one or both may have, such as mental illness or an addictive personality, you need to instruct the body that you need every emotional or mental disease corrected, which you can do rapidly via Sequential Healing, as described in Chapter 8.

Remote Healing

Correcting intolerances two people may have for each other may require you to do energy healing remotely on someone who is not your patient. If you are not comfortable working on someone with positive energy without their explicit permission, don't do it.

Every time I have chosen to work on someone without their explicit permission, I have had the permission of their significant other, parent, other close relative or friend. Afterward, their issue has always muscle-tested as corrected, and their lives became easier.

For example, Barbara L. contacted me about her son, who had been diagnosed as bipolar. He lived across the country from where my office is located, and, according to his mother, would never consciously agree to muscle testing. She asked me if I would work on him.

Having her permission to do so, I treated him long distance.

The following week, I asked her, "How is your son?"

"Oh, so much better!" she told me.

In this case, the man's mother was convinced I could help him, and I was glad to do so.

Distance healing is discussed more in Chapter 13.

"A Different Man"

Sandra R. came to see me for various diseases and musculoskeletal pains. After she experienced the energy healing that I performed on her, she became interested in correcting other conditions in her life.

She told me that she and her husband had been dealing with a lot of emotional issues in their marriage that had caused her to experience a great deal of strain. She said she was desperate and willing to do anything that could help.

The first thing I did was envision Sandra and her husband together. When muscle testing, her strong muscle weakened, indicating the two of them were currently incompatible in some manner. I took the same approach as if I was treating an intolerance to sugar, gluten or dairy products. I reset the muscle to strong, then tested for the primary emotional trigger that was responsible for the emotional intolerance.

Then I muscle tested and found the meridian that was being interfered with by the emotional trigger, and "streamed" the primary emotional trigger to the meridian pulse point, as you learned in Chapter 6.

I continued this procedure several times, correcting each primary emotional trigger the body indicated, until the muscle no longer weakened when I envisioned Sandra and her husband together.

Sandra returned to my office about a week later with a big grin on her face, as though she had just won the Lottery. She was so happy, she gave me a big hug and began to thank me and cry at the same time. She said her husband was "a different man," that he was calm for the first time since she had known him, and that he was no longer angry or critical of her.

This procedure can be life altering for many people. It can be employed for mother/daughter, father/son or sister/brother relationships, or any other interpersonal relationships.

Graduate Level

You can correct emotional intolerances by telling the body to go on autopilot and correct the intolerances sequentially, just as you can do with multi-layered diseases. The energy automatically flows to one or both people's bodies, in the order of most importance.

For example, say a husband is bipolar, and the Universe and the body both understand that this condition is the most important thing to correct, in order for the couple to become more tolerant of each other, and also for subsequent corrections to be more effective. The second most important thing to correct for this couple might be the wife's addiction; the third most important is the wife's depression, and so on.

It is highly possible that after these three most important issues are corrected, all of the couple's remaining emotional intolerances will be solved. It's just like the bowling ball example: When you strike the first pin accurately, all the remaining pins fall without any additional effort on your part.

Emotional Intolerances
Chapter Summary

1. When muscle testing for intolerances between people, envision the people together, and intend that if they are emotionally intolerant to each other, a strong muscle will weaken. Often there are multiple issues to correct.
2. Correcting emotional intolerances two people may have for each other may require you to do energy healing remotely on someone who is not your patient. If you are uncomfortable working on someone without their explicit permission, don't do it.
3. You can correct emotional intolerances by telling the body to go on autopilot and correct the intolerances sequentially, just as you can do with multi-layered diseases.

Chapter 11

Miscellaneous Intolerances

After treatments with my Energy Healing Unlocked system, most of my patients have rarely needed to return to my office. Instead, the vast majority returned to enjoying their lives.

But a small percentage have their symptoms return within a few hours, days or weeks. I have discovered three reasons for this: 1) They are reactivating the same or similar emotions that triggered their ailment; 2) They are highly sensitive people; or 3) They were intolerant to things I had not previously known about.

A person can become intolerant to anything. I've had patients who were intolerant to things like the wind, the moon, the stars, the sun, water, plastic, the clothes they were wearing, light, darkness, certain types of music, bell peppers, meat, even specific words. Anything you can think of, a person can become intolerant to. As with diseases and other ailments, the root cause is always emotions.

For purposes of this discussion, "intolerance" means your body does not like something. "Intolerance" encompasses hearing, seeing, smelling, touching, tasting or even simply thinking of something or someone that causes emotional or physical upset — even if this is not consciously known by the person.

An intolerance can create any number of unpleasant reactions. Allergies, for example, occur when the body releases the chemical histamine when exposed to something to which it is intolerant, typically creating a runny nose, watery eyes or difficulty breathing. An alcoholic may enjoy drinking vodka, but they may develop cirrhosis of the liver because their body has an intolerance to it.

How does someone become intolerant to bell peppers, cars or anything else that other people can handle easily? Usually because of an unpleasant, possibly horrible emotional association with that thing, experience, word or concept.

For example, if a child was punished for not eating everything on her plate by being required to sit in a chair for hours every day, that child could grow up to become an adult who has an unconscious aversion to chairs, a particular type of chair or even the word "chair."

Worse, if a child witnessed her sibling seriously injured in an automobile accident, once she becomes an adult, the mere concept of "car" could cause a daily overwhelm of her emotional system, without her consciously knowing.

Imagine being exposed daily, or possibly multiple times per day, to something that has always horrified you, whether consciously or not. Before long, your nervous system would become overloaded and stressed, generating myriad types of symptoms. Years of this can create conditions like high blood pressure or even diseases such as cancer, due to continual imbalanced energy in the body.

When you have a patient for whom no correction seems to be holding, don't give up. Test them for miscellaneous intolerances.

Correcting miscellaneous intolerances is done using the same techniques taught earlier in this book: Muscle test to discover the primary emotional triggers, locate the affected meridian pulse point(s) on their wrist(s), then make the correction.

Wind Intolerance

Intolerance to the wind is a condition known as ancraophobia, and alternately as anemophobia. Many people feel worse on windy days, and some research indicates that suicide rates increase during windy conditions.

When I discover via muscle testing that a person is physically or emotionally intolerant to the wind, I will say to them, "You don't like the wind, do you?" They are always relieved — and a little surprised — that I know this without them having specifically told me. I will blow on their ankle to represent wind, then muscle test. When their previously-strong muscle weakens so dramatically that I can use my little finger to collapse it, I know it is true.

Who knows what can cause people to become intolerant to something as natural on this Earth as the wind, or for others to become intolerant to the full moon. It's not for us to understand, but rather for us to know that we can restore our patients to balance, regardless of their symptoms or causes.

Test Both Emotional and Physical

When helping patients overcome intolerances that fall into the "Miscellaneous" category, you must muscle test for both emotional and physical effects. For example, one person may muscle test positive only for emotional effects as a result of their intolerance, while another may have developed physical issues, as well.

Word Intolerances

Some patients whose conditions return frequently can be intolerant to words. Yes, words! How can this be? By their association of a word or words with a person, an emotional event or period of time in their lives.

Words have the real capability to create emotional upsets that overload some people. If a person is bombarded daily with words they don't know they have an intolerance to, nothing we can do for them will remain corrected, unless and until we also correct their intolerances to those words. For example, it is easy to understand that a person could become upset at the mere mention of the word "cancer," based upon their own experiences.

But via muscle testing, I have also encountered intolerances to seemingly-benign words such as "good." This was confusing to me at first, but I figured the body knew what it was doing. When I muscle-tested the concept of "good" for that particular patient, I learned that, whether unconsciously or consciously, she had become uncomfortable when someone was nice. I asked her if she was suspicious of people who were extra kind to her, like if someone did a favor for her. She said yes, that she definitely becomes suspicious if someone is nice to her, wondering what their ulterior motive is. She said she always feels like asking them, "What do you want from me?"

Sometimes patients will say things like, "I just don't feel like living," "Everything just seems to upset me," or, "I just feel like a loser and that I am worthless," but they cannot explain why. They usually say they don't feel under any unusual emotional stress other than an underlying feeling of something being "off" 24 hours a day. This can be caused by word intolerances, being exposed to words the mind and body have come to believe are harmful.

To muscle test for word intolerances, think "Abnormal issue" with the word you think is at the root cause of the patient's emotional reaction, while expecting the strong muscle to weaken if the patient has an abnormal issue with that word. If the muscle weakens, reset it to strong, then proceed with your testing and correcting as previously described.

Alternately, once you become adept enough, you can instruct the body to correct word intolerances via Sequential Healing on autopilot. To determine when the body is done making its corrections, muscle test for "Word Intolerances" again. When the muscle remains strong, the body is signaling that it has completed its process.

You can test for word intolerances at any time during the course of your treatment, but I usually only test for them when I have a patient whose symptoms inexplicably continue to return frequently.

Highly Sensitive People

When you have a patient who is intolerant to many things such as the wind, plastics, the sun or multiple words, you have a highly sensitive and emotional patient. Their bodies have become so emotionally overloaded, that almost anything upsets their balance.

When I recognize this in a patient, whether they are male or female, and tell them they are highly sensitive and emotional, I usually reach for a tissue for them. Simply acknowledging their sensitivity makes them feel understood in a way they rarely are, and they usually begin to cry. They often say, "Finally someone understands me and is going to help me."

Larry N.

Word intolerances can be tricky to uncover. Here's a good example of how I discovered what to correct for a young man named Larry N.

Larry lived with his mother, Melanie, across the country from where my office is, so I performed my treatments remotely, over the telephone, using a surrogate's arm. (Distance Healing is explained in Chapter 13.)

I asked Melanie to send me a list of Larry's symptoms so I could have them in front of me when I began treatment. However, when her email arrived, I noticed she sent me the list of her son's symptoms in letter form, describing how he acted and reacted to his daily routine in a story-like manner. This recounting of his daily routine, physical symptoms and emotional idiosyncrasies was quite long. To save time, I decided to test line by line, telling the body that if there was a symptom or intolerance in any particular line, the muscle would weaken. As I tested, every line in her story caused a muscle to weaken, so I had to test one word at a time.

In her story, Melanie described Larry going downstairs into the basement to get eggs for breakfast. On the way, his mind wandered so much, that he forgot why he went to the basement. This was a common occurrence for Larry.

Via muscle testing, the words "stairs," "basement," "eggs," "forgot" and "him" caused the muscle I was testing to weaken on his behalf.

I couldn't possibly know the reason Larry had developed an intolerance to each of those words, but I simply performed corrections on each word.

Melanie advised me that as a result of the treatment, Larry began not only to feel better about going downstairs and to remember things without getting confused, but he also began to improve in other areas of his life. Additionally, Melanie said that Larry's physical symptoms and other emotional issues abated.

Katie P.

Katie P. was a highly sensitive patient. I treated her remotely because she lived a couple states away from my office. I corrected her bipolar disorder, depression and anxiety. I also corrected all of her food intolerances that I could find, her self-intolerances (see Chapter 12), her allergies and autoimmune disorders.

Muscle testing indicated these dysfunctions were corrected, and she said she felt much improved, but symptoms that mimicked those conditions kept returning frequently.

Over a period of time it became difficult to make any corrections for her that could last longer than a few hours. As her condition worsened, her mental state followed, to the point she could no longer spend time around people without her symptoms becoming even worse.

She was feeling so horrible, that she actually began giving things away, in preparation for her death.

Then I remembered Melanie and her son, Larry. I asked Katie to email me what I jokingly referred to as a "manifesto" of her daily routine and her early life in synopsis form. I told her to start at the beginning of her life and write all the good and bad she felt comfortable telling me about.

When I received Katie's several pages of writing, I began muscle testing one sentence at a time. Every sentence caused weakening of a strong muscle.

Then I began testing for individual words. I had anticipated certain nouns and verbs would cause weakening of a strong muscle, and they did, but what I had not anticipated was that words like "run," "stairs," "awake," "school," "door," "closet," "clothes," "bed," "television" and "food," also did. I corrected them all.

After about 20 minutes of this procedure, Katie told me she was feeling much better, so I continued making corrections to any word that caused a strong muscle to weaken, no matter how insignificant or small it seemed. Words like "it," "me," "was," "not," "one," "afraid," "alone," "as," "began," and "answer," also caused weakness while I was muscle testing. Only the patient's body knew what this meant, but I corrected those as well.

After a week, Katie said she not only felt much better, but actually felt for the first time in a long time that she wanted to live.

After treating Katie in this manner for a handful more times, all of her physical and emotional symptoms disappeared.

New Person Entirely

Crystal S. had a number of emotional and physical issues that responded well to my initial treatment that I provided to her remotely. But after a couple of days, her symptoms began returning. I treated her again, and once again, the majority of her symptoms returned within a few hours to a few days.

When I asked Crystal about her daily personal life, she said she was living with a man who was abusive to her, to the point that she feared for her life if she ever attempted to end the relationship.

She was convinced that her boyfriend would never agree to treatment using energy healing, and asked if I could treat him remotely, too.

(Treating a patient's friend, relative or significant other remotely will require you to perform energy work on someone who is not your patient. If you are not comfortable working on someone without their explicit permission, don't do it. In my personal experience, every time I have chosen to do so, both people's lives have become better.)

After I did my first remote treatment of Crystal's boyfriend, she said his behavior improved for the remainder of the day, but the following day his abrasive and abusive attitude returned.

I suggested to Crystal that she email me his daily routine and the attitudes she usually experienced from him throughout the day. Once I received her email, I began muscle testing for word intolerances. I discovered that every other word I tested, caused a muscle to weaken.

After the first time I treated her boyfriend for word intolerances, Crystal said she noted a significant change in his behavior, that he seemed much happier and less critical of her. After my third treatment of him, Crystal said his behavior had changed so much he was actually pleasant to be around, nice and "cuddly" toward her, and that he had not been this way to her for years. She described him as a "new person entirely."

"What He Said"

Many times a patient will attempt to explain a physical feeling or an emotional issue but they have difficulty describing it, or at times their symptoms are so vague and complicated, it is difficult to figure out where to start and what to test. The best way to handle this is by testing and correcting using one or both of these methods:

1. Write keywords of what the patient describes and muscle test those words. If a strong muscle weakens, make the corrections. For example, while the patient is talking to me, I might write: "jittery, confused, no energy, exhausted, tired, scared, can't remember anything." Then I look at the words I wrote and muscle test each word individually. If the muscle weakens, the body is signaling there is an issue that needs correcting. Correct it as described in Chapter 6.

2. When a patient gives too much information, is vague or does not stop talking for awhile and you cannot write down everything they say due to the volume of information, simply write the words, "What he said," or "What she said." Then hold the feeling of what the person just said, and muscle test. When you muscle test, the muscles will weaken. Continue testing and correcting until the muscle no longer weakens to the concept of "What he/she said."

This concept might sound crazy, but it works. The Universe knows what he or she said.

Pain

What can you do for a patient who experiences disabling pain, but for whom all MRIs, X-rays and other tests indicate nothing is wrong? Test them for "pain."

Think of the concept of the pain the patient is describing, and, while muscle testing, expect the body to weaken a strong muscle if there is pain. If the muscle weakens, reset the muscle to strong. Then muscle test for the primary emotional trigger, then for the meridian pulse point(s) being affected by the emotion(s), resetting the muscle to strong after every response that weakens it.

Correct the dysfunction by "streaming" that primal emotion to the meridian pulse point(s) on the patient's wrists, as described in Chapter 6. Or, if the body indicates via muscle testing that it's allowable, go straight to the heart.

Energy Fine Tuning

Every part of our bodies has energy flowing through it, so if someone's energy is imbalanced, deficient or too high, they may feel "off," or "just not themselves." Muscle test for the concept of energy imbalance. If there is an issue, correct it as you have done with other issues, as described earlier in this book.

Correcting energy imbalance is what I call "fine tuning." It is best used in difficult cases in which a person's body does not respond as readily as others, or for a person who is normally healthy, who may have allowed a circumstance to upset their balance.

Nutritional Deficiencies & Digestion

Why can some people eat nothing but junk food, sodas, beer, potato chips and candy for years, and live for a long time without any apparent harmful results, while other people who stick to healthy diets become ill?

People who can eat junk food most of the time and remain relatively healthy, are those whose bodies are functioning relatively normally. (I am not recommending junk food, by any means.)

However, when our emotions have gotten us out of balance, our bodies lose their capacities to function at their maximum abilities. When this happens, taking various dietary supplements is not as effective as most people wish, until the cause of their nutritional deficiencies is corrected.

> *Emotions are almost always responsible for bodies being unable to absorb or process nutrients, minerals and supplements.*

By using muscle testing, you can uncover the reason a body is unable to digest properly or sufficiently absorb the nutrients from the foods they are eating:

1. Begin with a strong muscle.
2. Think "All nutritional deficiencies," and expect the muscle to weaken if the body is nutritionally deficient. Reset the muscle to strong.
3. Muscle test for the primary emotional trigger(s), resetting the muscle to strong after each response that weakens it.
4. Find the associated meridian pulse point(s), or go straight to the heart, if the body will allow it.
5. Put the body on autopilot to correct them all.
6. Retest to confirm your results.

Answers Will Come

Please do not take my word for anything I have written in this book. Instead, become an expert muscle-tester. Ask the body, test and correct for yourself. You will be amazed, as I have been, with the physical and emotional issues you are able to help patients' bodies heal from, using my Energy Healing Unlocked system.

Being unable to easily find or understand how to help someone does not mean their ailment is incurable. It simply means we have to become more creative in our muscle testing, question asking and solution seeking. Keep asking whatever higher power you believe in how you can help your patients. Answers will come.

Miscellaneous Intolerances
Chapter Summary

1. Correcting miscellaneous intolerances is done using the same techniques taught earlier in this book: muscle testing to discover the primary emotional triggers, locating the affected meridian pulse point(s) on the patient's wrist(s), then making the correction(s). Go straight to the heart, if the body allows it.
2. A person can become intolerant to anything, including the moon, wind, light, darkness, certain types of music, bell peppers, meat, even specific words.
3. A person can become intolerant to something that other people typically handle easily because of an unpleasant, possibly horrible, emotional association with that thing, experience, word or concept.
4. When helping patients overcome intolerances that fall into the "Miscellaneous" category, you must muscle test for both emotional and physical effects.

Chapter 12

Self-Intolerance

One of the most prevalent, destructive and generally unrecognized intolerances I have discovered is what I call, "Self-Intolerance." Yes, that means intolerance to oneself, or to an aspect of oneself.

Self-Intolerance is similar to autoimmune diseases in that the body begins responding abnormally to a normal body part or function, such as its own blood, skin, bones, brain, muscles, organs or to the person's own thoughts.

But with Self-Intolerance, it isn't antibodies turning against the person's body. The person's emotions have created the physical dysfunction. Just as with autoimmune conditions, Self-Intolerance continues to worsen if not stopped.

The body has also indicated via muscle testing that a fetus, while in the womb, can be intolerant to itself. (A fetus is affected by the mother's emotions.)

One of your clues that a patient suffers from Self-Intolerance, is if they have symptoms that mimic those of well-known diseases, such as a person who has a sensitivity to wheat or sugar, when laboratory blood tests show they do not have Celiac disease or diabetes.

In either scenario, patients can take normal actions associated with keeping symptoms of those ailments under control, such as reducing wheat or sugar in their diet, and they will feel better. However, if the true cause is Self-Intolerance, the symptoms will continue to worsen over time and/or cease responding to earlier corrective measures.

Self-Intolerance is corrected via the eight primary emotional triggers.

Correcting Self-Intolerance

Fortunately, correcting Self-Intolerance is done the same way we correct other ailments.

Here is a sample muscle testing script for correcting Self-Intolerance:

1. Begin with a strong muscle. Think or say, "Self-Intolerance," while muscle testing. If the person has Self-Intolerance, the muscle will weaken.

2. Reset the muscle to strong.

3. Muscle test for the primary emotional trigger and perform the correction as described in Chapter 6.

4. Next, because most people who have Self-Intolerance have multiple instances of it, place the body on Autopilot, telling it to correct all Self-Intolerance sequentially.

5. Continue muscle-testing until the body signals via a strong muscle that all instances of Self-Intolerance have been corrected, remembering to reset the muscle to strong after each response that weakens it.

It is paramount that you are thinking the concept of "Self Intolerance" while muscle testing, otherwise the body can begin correcting other intolerances such as gluten, dairy, etc., which in itself could be a great service to your patient, but would still leave their Self-Intolerance uncorrected.

Wanda

Wanda had numerous health conditions including Type 2 diabetes and headaches. She had been advised by her physician that she had gout, and indeed she had classic symptoms of gout including "Hammer Toe," bunion deformity and pain in her large toe.

She also complained of feeling very sick after eating or drinking anything sweet, and also that for many years she'd had to drink water very slowly or else she felt sick afterward.

Many of Wanda's symptoms disappeared with my initial energy treatments. But some of them returned frequently, which annoyed both of us.

The conventional thinking is that a high level of uric acid indicates gout, but the results of a blood test Wanda's physician ordered showed her uric acid levels were normal.

Similarly, a high blood glucose level can indicate diabetes. Wanda's diabetes symptoms were so severe, I suspected her blood glucose level would be over 200 milligrams per deciliter, but her test results were 112, only slightly elevated.

I was stumped. Then I had a hunch.

I had Wanda touch her hair and skin and muscle tested each. Her strong muscle weakened each time. Then I began thinking "Wanda's blood," "Wanda's fat," "Wanda's muscles," and so on, and muscle-tested each one. Once again, her muscle weakened every time, indicating she was intolerant to everything in her body, including her own uric acid. This is how I came to understand the concept of Self-Intolerance.

I began my correction as I would with every other ailment, disease or pain. I identified the primary emotional trigger, then identified the meridian pulse point affected by the emotion. To make sure everything her body had become intolerant to was corrected, I placed her body on autopilot and instructed it to correct sequentially all that needed to be corrected.

After just one treatment none of Wanda's symptoms returned. In addition, she no longer felt sick after eating sugar, she had more energy and greater mental clarity. Lastly, she no longer feels sick after drinking water, no matter how fast she drinks it. Her life changed.

Since Wanda, Self-Intolerance is one of the first things I test on my patients.

Self-Intolerance
Chapter Summary

1. Self-Intolerance is intolerance to oneself or to an aspect of oneself, in which the body begins responding abnormally to a normal body part or function, such as one's own blood, skin, bones, brain, muscles, organs or even thoughts.
2. Self-Intolerance can be corrected by going through the normal list of eight primary emotional triggers and correction procedures, as described in earlier chapters.

Chapter 13

Distance Healing

When I have a patient who is physically unable to handle muscle testing without discomfort, I ask them to bring a healthier person with them, such as their spouse or a friend, and I will muscle test using that surrogate's arm. The techniques in this book are equally as accurate using a surrogate's muscle for testing.

Eventually I began to ask myself, "If I can muscle test and treat a patient from inches away, how far can I be from them and still correct their dysfunctions?" I wondered if energy healing was like Wi-Fi signals, and if so, how far can our signals reach?

To find out, I decided to try correcting dysfunctions and diseases on friends and relatives who had no knowledge of my testing, nor who even knew that I did anything other than adjusting people's spines, as conventional chiropractors do.

I chose friends and relatives who had chronic ailments such as migraine headaches, allergies, rheumatoid arthritis and plantar fasciitis, and whom I knew would not mind me correcting their conditions. I did not tell any of them about my experiment until I was done.

Using my wife's arm as the muscle-testing surrogate, I performed the entire testing and healing procedure just as I would have done if they had been there in front of me.

I waited two weeks to give them all time to notice a difference in how they were feeling. Then I called each one on the phone, ostensibly just to chat. Somewhere in the middle of our conversation, I would ask something like, "Hey, Reba, how are your allergies doing?" or "Hey, Bud, how is your plantar fasciitis doing?" Without exception, EVERY one of these friends and relatives had similar responses: "You know, now that you mention it, it hasn't bothered me in a couple of weeks."

I could only stare in disbelief as I got off each one of these phone calls. I was astounded!

Energy flow is not constrained by physical boundaries. You can direct healing energy anywhere.

Soon, I began accepting referrals from my current patients to help their relatives and friends who live all around the planet. I treated them remotely and got the same results as I did with patients who were right in front of me in my office.

This has proven so helpful to people, that about 50 percent of my practice has become distance healing, some of which I do while on the phone, so I can explain my findings to them.

Making Corrections Remotely

When you are doing distance healing, making corrections is almost identical to when a patient is right in front of you, with the minor exception that you are using a surrogate's arm for muscle testing, with the intent that the surrogate's arm is answering for your patient's body. Simply shift your focus from the surrogate sitting in front of you, to the person you are treating.

You do not need to have a photograph
of the person you are treating,
nor do you need to meet them in person beforehand
for distance healing to be effective.

Merely visualize the concept of the other person, then do your testing using the surrogate's arm, as described earlier.

Remember, muscles weaken and strengthen during muscle testing based on *your* thought process about your patient's situation, regardless of how far from you the patient is located, and also regardless whose arm you are using to do your muscle testing.

Using my Energy Healing Unlocked system to perform healing from any distance is blessedly simple:

Be in a quiet room where you will have no interruptions. Muscle test, as instructed in prior chapters, while thinking of the patient. Test for the patient's primary emotional trigger(s), then test their meridian pulse points along their wrists one by one, while saying aloud, or thinking of their primary emotional trigger(s) and each of their pulse points, as you have learned in prior chapters. Or go straight to the heart if their body will allow it.

It may take awhile before you are sensitive enough to feel the energy as the corrections are being made. Trust that it is working, and muscle test using the surrogate's arm to confirm.

Can you see the phenomenal tool you now possess?

Distance Healing
Chapter Summary

1. If a patient is physically unable to handle muscle testing without discomfort, you can use a healthier person's arm as a surrogate for your muscle testing. It is equally accurate.

2. You can use a surrogate's arm to muscle test and correct conditions for someone at a distance. You do not need to have a photograph of the person you are treating, nor do you need to meet them in person beforehand.

3. Energy flow is not constrained by physical boundaries. You can direct healing energy anywhere.

Chapter 14

Tips for Chiropractors

As chiropractors, we have been taught that the misalignment of vertebrae is what creates our patients' ailments, and that spinal adjustments help our patients get better. I believe this.

However, don't most of your patients need to keep returning to your office for the same, or similar, adjustments?

As chiropractors, we even place them on "Maintenance Care" programs so they will return once a month for many months, or even for the rest of their lives.

Are we hoping to get different results by doing the same thing over and over again?

Thinking the fault lies within our patients' vertebrae
is like building a brick wall,
then blaming the bricks if the wall collapses.
What caused the bricks to lose support?

After practicing my Energy Healing Unlocked system for some years, I no longer believe that spinal misalignment is the root cause of our patients' health issues. I'm not saying that vertebrae can't become misaligned. They do, and standard chiropractic adjustments help.

In human bodies, a myriad of things can cause vertebrae to misalign, including supporting structures, ligaments, tendons, muscles, discs, cartilage, inflammation or arthritis.

And emotions.

In chiropractic, we are taught merely to realign the vertebrae. How do you, as a chiropractor, gain access to, and provide healing for your patients' other body parts? By using my Energy Healing Unlocked system, as explained in this book.

When you are beginning, I recommend having a list of every muscle, ligament, tendon, disc, type of inflammation, arthritis and autoimmune disease in front of you, related to the part of the body you are correcting. Muscle test and correct until the body signals via muscle testing (with a strong muscle remaining strong), that you have finished.

Remember to test for and correct the concept of "pain."

As you become more proficient, you will be able to use my Sequential Healing and Autopilot techniques, as described in Chapter 8. Soon you will be able to make corrections in minutes, with very few follow-up visits.

Using my Energy Healing Unlocked techniques, you will be able to help more people than ever before.

Tips for Chiropractors
Chapter Summary

1. We chiropractors have been taught that the misalignment of vertebrae causes our patients' ailments. In most human bodies, emotions are the root cause of vertebral misalignment.
2. We can correct the root causes of misalignments by using my Energy Healing Unlocked system, especially my Sequential Healing and Autopilot techniques.

Chapter 15

The Power of Joy

*Joy does not simply happen to us.
We have to choose joy and
keep choosing it every day.*

— *Henri J. M. Nouwen*

As I continue to correct more and more emotional causes of different diseases, ailments and dysfunctions in my practice, I am struck by the fact that people who have a positive outlook on life are much healthier than those who are emotionally negative, sad, angry, grieving, and those who won't let go of the past.

Have you ever wondered why some people's cancer returns? Or why others carry their symptoms and ailments throughout their lives? The emotional triggers that caused their issues in the first place are being re-introduced in some form or another via the choices they make.

Long-lasting healing of emotional-based illnesses is similar to the success of a person who has chosen to diet and embark on an exercise program, and who has lost 50 or 100 pounds. When they continue exercising and eating healthily, the weight stays off. However, if they stop exercising and return to eating cheeseburgers, potato chips and drinking soda pop five days per week, the weight will come right back on.

For a person to remain healthy after energy healing, they need to strengthen their new emotional foundation. This can mean ceasing old, harmful patterns of behavior, or removing themselves from unhealthy situations. The situations might not be identical to the ones that created their dysfunction, however, they may trigger similar emotional responses.

For example, when we experience highly charged emotions with a spouse or significant other, frequent run-ins with a relative, continual stress at work, or constantly feel like we never have enough time, we create primary emotional triggers.

As humans, we also create emotional triggers through our thought processes. For example, have you ever told yourself any of the following:

"I'm not good enough."
"I'm unlovable."
"I'm unhealthy."

If we believe those thoughts, or anything similar, we aren't able to allow alternative, healthier emotions into our bodies.

> *Anything negative we believe about ourselves harms our bodies.*

Try this for yourself: Imagine you are furious at your boss. You are spitting mad because your salary increase, the one you have been promised for two years, was given to someone with less experience and seniority than you have. Set this book down, close your eyes and ponder that thought for five seconds, but no more.

Notice how merely reading this brief tale of injustice caused your body to feel different? You may have started clenching your jaw or making a fist. Your heart rate increased, or maybe you felt a burning in your heart, imperceptibly at first, then more, the longer you thought about the situation.

Multiply that by the amount of anger and frustration many of us subject ourselves to daily. Imagine how hard your body works to combat those negative effects.

So what is the best tool available to keep ourselves in balance, while continuing to lead our normal lives?

Joy.

When feeling joy, bodily organs begin returning to their normal functionality, and other conditions begin to clear up, seemingly like magic. The longer we can sustain our joyful moods, the more time our bodies have to heal.

*F*eelings of joy change our body chemistry.

Once we get into the habit of living in joy, it becomes easy.

One of the most important gifts we can bestow upon our patients is the knowledge that they are in control of their own healing and future health.

This is a revolutionary concept for most people.

Robert and Winona

Here's one of the most beautiful illustrations of the power of joy I know.

Robert was diagnosed with a brain tumor. He saw the tumor on his CT scan results. He and his doctor talked about treatment, but Robert's plan was to retire from his 35-year career and move to a city 5,000 miles away from his home, so he could die without becoming a burden to his children. At the time, he was unmarried.

During one of his hospital visits, he met a lovely woman washing dishes at a concession stand. They soon began dating, and fell in love.

One year later, Robert returned to the hospital. His doctor sat in amazement, as he compared, side-by-side, the results of Robert's most recent brain scan, with the one from the prior year.

The tumor was clearly visible in the earlier scan. In the most recent scan, the tumor was completely gone. Robert had not undergone surgery, chemotherapy or radiation, nor was he taking any medications.

"It looked as if someone or something had dug the tumor right out of me," Robert said.

The only "treatment" he had undergone was to experience tremendous joy. That allowed his body to return to functioning normally. It dissolved the tumor naturally, without outside intervention.

Robert and his wife continue to live together in joy. Twenty years later, the tumor has not returned.

Joy Techniques for your Patients

Entire books are filled with concepts of living in joy, so I will provide you only brief examples of what I advise my patients. For some people, being introduced to the power of joy by a doctor is strong enough medicine that patients happily delve into the topic more deeply on their own.

Focal Points

Find joy in areas of your life that do not involve your stress points. It's much easier to find joy in your dog's delight at your return home, a beautiful flower or your adorable grandchild, than in a cancer diagnosis.

This is not to discount a cancer diagnosis, nor the associated trauma, whatsoever. It is merely shifting your focal point to happier topics on a more frequent basis.

Make 'Em Laugh

Anything that makes you laugh is extraordinarily powerful. I typically tell my patients to watch comedy movies, humorous television shows and funny animal videos.

Positive Affirmations

Recite positive affirmations that are meaningful to you. Words generate emotional responses, so they are much more powerful than most people realize. Choose from the examples below, or create ones that are meaningful to you. There are books upon books filled with positive affirmations.

"I am worthy of being loved."
"I am fortunate."
"I am happy."
"I am generous."
"I reach out with forgiveness."
"It is in God's hands."
"I am grateful to be alive."

If you choose to devote the time, you may muscle test your patients to discover which positive affirmations are most healing to them. Many patients will instantaneously recognize which ones are most powerful for themselves, simply by saying each one aloud and noting how they feel.

Self-Appreciation

The more we acknowledge we are worthy human beings, the easier it is for our bodies to heal. As with the affirmations above, choose from the examples below, or create new ones that have meaning to you.

"I am a loving, caring, beautiful person inside and out."
"I am a good wife/mother/husband/father/boyfriend/girlfriend."
"I do the best I know how to do."
"I believe in myself."

Happy Thoughts

When I previously dwelled on negative things in my life, my wife allowed me to vent for a few minutes, but then would begin exclaiming, "Happy Thoughts! Happy Thoughts!" Honestly, at first I was annoyed by this. But I soon realized her wisdom.

Only harm comes to our bodies from wallowing in anything other than happy thoughts. When we become aware and disciplined enough to shift our focus from lamenting, to more pleasurable thoughts, our minds become reprogrammed to become the joy-seeking vehicles we are meant to be.

Many of my patients have told me they have tried various methods of positive thinking, but did not see or feel immediate results. Creating joy in your life is similar to planting a garden. Don't abandon your garden simply because your seeds don't sprout overnight. Continue watering and tending your garden, while simultaneously seeking support from your healing community of choice.

Life is designed to be simple, easy and fun.

You may believe this all sounds too simple. But remember, you also probably thought energy healing was going to be harder than it is, until reading this book.

May you go forth in the best of health and success in treating your patients — or maybe yourself — using my Energy Healing Unlocked system.

Let us go out and heal the world!

The Power of Joy
Chapter Summary

1. People who have a positive outlook on life are much healthier than those who are emotionally negative, sad, angry, grieving, and those who won't let go of the past.
2. For a person to remain healthy after energy healing, they need to strengthen their new emotional foundation.
3. Feelings of joy change our body chemistry.

Want to Learn More?

There is so much more I can explain in person than can easily be contained in this book, including additional techniques I have developed since this book was written.

Please contact me if you are interested in learning more. I love teaching and sharing my latest discoveries, so more people can regain their health and vitality.

Please reach me through my website:
www.EnergyHealingUnlocked.com

Glossary

Applied Kinesiology — The premise that touching an area of the body triggers energies that cause muscles to either weaken or strengthen.

Chi — Energy.

Chiropractor — A doctor who realigns vertebrae.

Correction — The removal, via Energy Healing Unlocked technique, of emotional influences that created an imbalance in a body.

Distance Healing — The ability to heal energetically without being in physical proximity.

Dysfunction — Less than perfect function; normally caused in the body by an imbalance.

Electromagnetic Frequencies — Computers, fluorescent lights, mobile phones, satellites, the moon, the sun, solar flares, wind gusts and so on.

Emotions — Anger, fear, sadness, joy, shame and so on; the root cause of all of our illnesses.

Glands — Structures in the body that regulate physical functions, collectively part of the endocrine system. The major glands are the hypothalamus, pituitary, thyroid, parathyroids, adrenals, pineal, and the reproductive organs.

Gluten — Substance found in wheat and certain flours.

Immediate Cause — The most recent or adjacent cause of something.

Intolerance — Sensitivity to emotion, food, object, person, word or other phenomenon, such as wind, that creates an emotional and/or physical imbalance in the body.

Joy — Happiness. Living in joy allows the body to become, or remain, healthy.

Kinesiology — The study of movement and motion.

Meridians — Channels in the body through which energy flows.

Muscle Testing — Technique of testing for a change in the strength of a patient's muscle that indicates that whatever you are testing either is (or is not) harmful to, or causing a dysfunction in your patient's body.

Neurolymphatic Reflexes — Areas in the body that encourage lymphatic drainage.

Organs — Structures that conduct functions in the body; the five vital organs are the brain, heart, liver, lungs and kidneys.

Pectoralis major (clavicular division) — Muscle in the front chest that connects to the front shoulder; commonly used for muscle testing.

Primal Cause — The root cause.

Primary Emotional Trigger — The root emotion that causes dysfunction in the body.

Pulse Points — Energy points on the inside of each wrist.

Qi — Energy.

Quadriceps — Muscle in the front of the thigh which can be used for muscle testing.

Reflex Points — Places on the body that, when touched, cause organs or muscles to have a reflex action.

Self-Intolerance — Intolerance to oneself or to an aspect of oneself.

Sequential Categorizing — The grouping of things into categories, then testing those categories sequentially.

Sequential Healing — Asking the body to heal in the order of most importance.

Structures — Bones, ligaments, tendons, muscles, teeth and sutures.

Sutures — Where two bones in the skull come together.

Therapy Localization — Diagnostic procedure in which body parts or external items are muscle tested to determine if one is creating a dysfunction.

Two-Point Therapy Localization — Diagnostic procedure in which the relationship between body parts and/or external items is muscle tested, to determine if one is creating a dysfunction in the other.

Index

Multiple Personality Disorder: 36, 122

Muscle aches: 2

Muscle lock: 54, 57-58

Muscle testing: 2, 11, 13, 27, 29, 33, 36, 39-40, 43-52, 54, 56-61, 65, 67, 69-82, 84-85, 87-90, 93-98, 103-114, 116-117, 119-120, 125, 127-130, 133-134, 137-139, 141-143, 145-147, 149, 150-152, 154, 166-167

Neurolymphatic reflexes: 166

Nutritional: 141-142

Obsessive Compulsive Disorder: 37, 67

Organs: 39, 44, 55, 68, 88, 90, 145, 148, 157, 165-167

Over-sympathetic: 69, 74, 85, 93-94

Pain: 1-3, 22-32, 35-36, 38, 49, 64, 66-69, 78-79, 82-85, 88, 105, 109-110, 112, 128, 140-141, 147-148, 154

Pectoralis major (clavicular division): 48, 50-51, 54, 56, 61, 166

Physician: 11, 23, 25, 30, 36, 67, 78, 107, 116, 147

Plantar Fasciitis: 38, 67, 149-150

Primal cause: 63-67, 69, 166

Primary emotional trigger: 69-72, 74, 77-78, 80-85, 91-93, 95-98, 101, 103-106, 108-109, 111-112, 114, 116, 119-121, 126, 129, 133, 141-143, 146, 148, 151, 156, 166

Pulse points: 88-93, 95-98, 101, 103-106, 109, 111, 120-121, 151, 166

Qi: 87, 166

Quadriceps: 51-52, 57, 166

Reflex points: 44-45, 55, 167

Remote Healing, see also Distance Healing: 128

Respiratory disease: 38

Rheumatoid Arthritis: 51, 81, 105, 107, 149

Schizophrenia: 36

Sciatica: 69, 82

Self-Intolerance: 137, 145-148, 167

Sequential Categorizing: 167

Sequential Healing: 107, 109-112, 116, 127, 135, 154, 167

Shoulder: 48-49, 51-52, 61, 68, 109, 112, 166

Sinus infection: 3

Skin disease: 24, 38

Spiritual: 29, 69, 71, 79, 85, 93

Structures: 39, 45, 154, 165-167

Sugar: 36, 47, 56, 67, 79, 129, 145-146, 148

Sugar on the floor: 79

Suicide: 118-119, 133

Sutures: 45, 167

Tendons: 1, 45, 154, 167

Tensor fascia lata muscle: 51-53, 57

Therapy Localization: 45-46, 61, 167

Thyroid: 1, 64-65, 88, 165

Tumor: 38, 158

Two-Point Therapy Localization: 167

Universe: 16, 41, 104, 115, 130, 140

Wheat, wheat flour: 31-32, 34-35, 46-47, 57, 145-146, 166

Wheelchair: 27, 31

Wind intolerance: 133

Word intolerances: 134-136, 139

Made in the USA
Columbia, SC
29 March 2020